What other are saying

"Dr. Barboa's book is an incredible addition to any library for anyone who works with or loves an individual on the autism spectrum. Her experience, compassion, and wisdom come through in a dynamic way. Anyone who wants to truly understand the complexities of autism will be extremely well served by this book—a veritable GPS system on how to effectively educate and advocate on behalf of individuals with autism. Dr. Barboa is on the right track, one that is so important as more and more people are being recognized as having autism."

—Michael Kaufman, Ph.D.,
President and CEO, SESI
(Specialized Education Services, Inc.)

"This is a delightfully easily read, yet vitally important book, which should be read by every parent who suspects autism in their child. These autism moms have taken their personal experiences, combined with their educational expertise, to produce an up-to-date, 'Autism Bible' which parents will refer to again and again. A must read! Five stars!"

—Dayna Busch,
Editor/Publisher of the
Missouri Autism Report Magazine

"The author's combination of parents and professionals captures the essence of what parents need to know about autism and their young child."

—Rachel Coley,
Parent of child on the spectrum

"This book is a wonderful blend of parent and professional perspective and knowledge."

—Susan Henderson, MS,
Director of Burrell Autism Center.

"Dr. Barboa has helped readers embrace autism by gracefully guiding us into the daily world of families with loved ones on the autism spectrum. Sharing the emotional and individual landscapes she respectfully shows the realities of autism, guiding family and professional readers through many aspects. Like a pebble dropped in the water, the circles of complexities are illuminated with grace and respect. This is a worthy read for all, a place of compassionate beginning."

—Patricia Pike, MS, CCC,
Clinical Associate Professor Emeritus

"Just as people who have autism desensitize to the world, we (representing the world) have to desensitize to people who have autism. The anxiety of the unknown is present in both populations. The contributors to this book have bridged a gap by making autism a safe, beautiful and intriguing world. I sincerely thank you for helping the world love my children better."

—R. Christi Eads MS,CCC-SLP,
Parent of a child on the autism spectrum

"Parents could not ask for a better resource than this book. This book is as unique as the children it describes."

—Braxton Baker, CCC-SLP,
CEO, Innovative Therapy Solutions, LLC

"A beautiful book that made me both laugh with the authors and cry with them. I felt I had gained five new friends to support me in my journey with autism. I wish I had this book 15 years ago."

—Tina S.,
Mother of a child on the autism spectrum

"A well written book that is insightful and thought provoking. A 'must read' for parents and teachers working with children on the autism spectrum."

—Tammy Parker,
Mother of a child on the autism spectrum

"A practical and thought provoking book which I will share with my personal and professional friends."

—Dr. Kaye Peery,
Superintendent of Schools, (ret.)

"*Stars in Her Eyes* will be a wonderful resource to be able to share with parents at our child care center. It can often feel like you are all alone when your child is diagnosed with a learning disability (or learning difference as I prefer to call it). This book will help parents understand that their journey need not be a lonely one".

—Jennifer Hendrickson,
Director, Tremont United Methodist
Child Care Center,
Tremont, IL.

"As a first year teacher this book is a valuable tool to guide me toward providing the best services possible for my students. As I read it I had several "ah-ha" moments thinking about students I serve. I recommend this book to all teachers, paras and parents."

—Brittani Stephens,
First year teacher,
Neosho, Missouri.

"One of the most relevant books to date about children on the autism spectrum. Thank you for putting the *child* first, not the *autism*."

—Dixie Love, MS
Early childhood special education teacher.

Stars in Her Eyes

DR. LINDA BARBOA
with
ELIZABETH OBREY

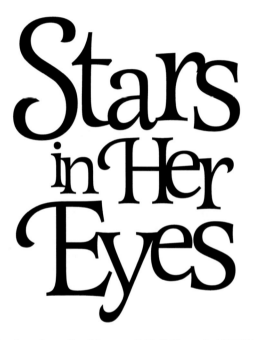

Stars in Her Eyes

Navigating the Maze of Childhood AUTISM

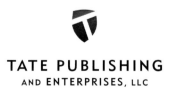

TATE PUBLISHING
AND ENTERPRISES, LLC

Published by Tate Publishing & Enterprises, LLC
127 E. Trade Center Terrace | Mustang, Oklahoma 73064 USA
1.888.361.9473 | www.tatepublishing.com

Tate Publishing is committed to excellence in the publishing industry. The company reflects the philosophy established by the founders, based on Psalm 68:11,
"The Lord gave the word and great was the company of those who published it."

Book design copyright © 2014 by Tate Publishing, LLC. All rights reserved.
Cover design by Jim Villaflores
Interior design by Mary Jean Archival

Published in the United States of America

ISBN: 978-1-63063-200-7
1. Family & Relationships / Autism Spectrum Disorders
2. Family & Relationships / General
14.02.04

Dedication

To my mother, Eunice Wainscott, and my husband Mike, for being the wind beneath my wings.

Acknowledgments

I would like to thank those who walked this path beside us, guiding us and giving encouragement while we gained the life experiences to write this book. My heartfelt appreciation to our parents, Floyd and Eunice Wainscott, David and JoAnne Stillwell, Randy, Kelley, and Eva Johnson.

I appreciate our spouses, Chuck, Gary, Patrick, Darren and Mike for always believing that we each had a message to share. Thanks to Muse Watson for convincing us that our message was important to others. Elise Mitchell added her experiences to several sections of the book and gave valuable insight. Heather Nicholson Photography patiently provided assistance with the pictures for the book.

Along with those who walked this path beside us, I thank those little people who we chased after over the years- Christopher, Courtney, Kyleigh, Nicole, Samantha, Brooke, Chase, Nathan, Joshuah, Izzy, Krista, Will, Kate, Becca, Carson, Kevin, Brian, Katie and Teddy. You filled our hearts with the knowledge that all children are special and deserve the best we have to give.

Special thanks to Elizabeth, Shelli, Jan and Sandy, the other four authors of this book. I thank you not only for the material you each provided but also for your friendship, spirit and attitude throughout the writing of the book. When I pulled this group together I told you all that it was important to me that we all still love each other when the book is completed. You made that part easy. I love you all.

About the Contributing Authors

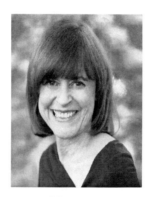

Mrs. Luck

Mrs. Jan Wainscott Luck holds a degree in speech pathology and audiology. She began her thirty-three year career with the State of Arkansas serving special needs clients from preschool age through adult in the day service center setting. For the last twenty-seven years she has been a public school speech therapist in Mt. Home, Arkansas where she has worked with children on the autism spectrum. She has mentored speech therapists that were new to the profession. Mrs. Luck has developed and presented continuing education seminars for teachers and therapists on the topic of autism.

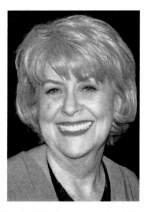

Sandy Nicholson (Mrs. Nic)

Mrs. Sandy Nicholson taught in public schools in kindergarten through third grade. She was also the owner-operator of a private preschool for many years and has been employed as a tutor for children with learning difficulties. She served as a mentor for nontenured teachers in her school district. She also trained student teachers from Bradley University. Mrs. Nicholson served on a local school board for 12 years, holding the office of president for two years. She has been an educator for thirty-two years and currently is a teacher in the infant/toddler program at Tremont United Methodist Child Care Center in Tremont, Illinois.

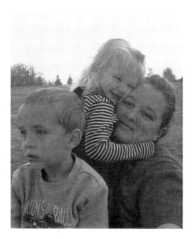

Shelli Allen with Joshuah and Izzy

Shelli has two children with autism—Joshuah, who is six years old and Israyel (Izzy), who is four. Both Josh and Izzy are nonverbal and attend a private school. Shelli serves as a mentor to parents of children with autism through the Sharing our Strengths Program in the State of Missouri. She has given presentations to teachers and parents on a variety of topics related to autism. Shelli is a consultant and advocate for essential oils.

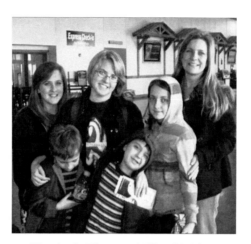
Elizabeth Obrey with Her Children

Elizabeth holds a degree in psychology. She is the mother of five children. The oldest, Nicole (age twenty-one), and the two youngest (Chase, age eight, and Nathan, age eleven) are on the spectrum. Brooke and Samantha are typically developing teenagers sandwiched between siblings on the spectrum. Chase and Nathan are currently enrolled in public schools. Nicole attends college in another state. Elizabeth is employed as a family advocate for ARC of the Ozarks. She has been a member of the Missouri Parent Advisory Committee on Autism and is the past president of Southwest Missouri Autism Network. Elizabeth is a member of the School, Family, Community Partnership and former owner of a business that promotes autism awareness. She was recently honored as one of Southwest Missouri's "10 Most Amazing Mothers" by Camp Barnabas.

Contents

Foreword

By Muse Watson

As an actor with a lifetime of movie and TV credits, I have played many roles. You may know me as a hook-wielding killer in the movie *I Know What You Did Last Summer*. Maybe you recognize me as a gentle, cat-loving convict named Charles Westmoreland from the television suspense drama series *Prison Break*. Many people know me as Special Agent Mike Franks, mentor to Jethro Gibbs on *NCIS*. From criminal to hero, I have played them all. Whether I am performing for stage, screen, or television, I study and prepare for each role meticulously.

But no role in my life has had more value or more meaning to me than my real life role of being a husband and father. This role, too, has required tremendous study and preparation. As my wife and I strive to provide everything needed for our daughter who is on the autism spectrum, we have found this goal to be time intensive and, at times, frustrating. Like other parents, we have searched for answers while trying to reach a goal that we have discovered is often a moving target.

I have come to a point on this journey where I feel that one of the most important things that we as parents can do to support each other is to share our experiences. Each of us may not have all of the answers (or maybe we don't even know the questions!). As we band together to share our successes and our frustrations, we all gain strength. This book offers families support and hope in nurturing and understanding children with autism.

I am excited to introduce *Stars in Her Eyes* as a practical, inspiring book, written to guide parents as they raise children on the autism spectrum. This book is well organized, covers a wide range of critical topics, and is enjoyable to read. As it was written by a group of parents and teachers, the reader will have the benefit of seeing both perspectives. The stories they add in each section bring the information to life and put a real life face on each topic.

I recommend *Stars in Her Eyes* not only for parents and teachers, but for anyone wanting to know more about this growing population.

Introduction

Dr. B: "You have a healthy baby boy!" The words ring like church bells in the ears of new parents. But a child's life does not always follow the roadmap created in the parents' hearts. Small nagging signs give way to larger, scarier symptoms. Then the dreaded words, "Your child has autism." These words echo in their heads like a freight train blasting through their hopes and dreams. Their minds race through a myriad of questions and their hearts begin to prematurely mourn what might have been. This is a moment that forever defines their family life. Despite the rapidly surging rate of autism, they feel alone.

Questions flood their minds. They face an overwhelming search for educational, medical, and social information. This search is complicated by conflicting information, unfamiliar vocabulary, and dizzying acronyms.

My career as a speech-language pathologist and an educator took me along a winding path as a public school special education director, university professor, owner of a private school, and director of an autism center.

During my tenure as director of the Rivendale Center for Autism, I became painfully aware that many parents were searching for practical advice. I also learned that many parents feel very alone when faced with this diagnosis. Mr. Muse Watson, star of stage, movies, and TV, happened to be performing a Christmas show in Branson last year and graciously came to spend an evening talking with the parents and teachers at Rivendale. He told of some of his experiences as the parent of a child on the spectrum. He shared things he has learned along the way and talked of continuing challenges. Throughout his presentation, his love for his daughter was shining through. By reaching out to tell us what he has learned from his daughter, he inspired us to do the same for others. He challenged us to share with others what we have learned on our journey and assure them they are not alone.

This book is a collection of practical suggestions to help the reader make it through the day-to-day challenges that autism presents. The contributing authors all have meaningful experiences with children with autism and want to share what they have learned over the years. To respect privacy and maintain confidentiality, some names and locations discussed in the book have been changed. As every child is a distinct individual, what works for one may not work for another. Your child's program will be developed by his team and will be based on his needs.

Mrs. Luck: When I was in college, autism was a fascinating topic to study but a very rare diagnosis. Throughout my years teaching special education, the prevalence skyrocketed to where it is today. I never really set my career path to become known as an autism resource; that just sort of evolved. My goal was to be a provider of special education services in the area of speech-language pathology. As the identification of students with autism grew, I found myself learning so much from these children. I am happy to share what they have taught me over the years.

Mrs. Nic: Coming from the mainstream classrooms, I look at the topic of autism from the perspective of a "regular education" teacher. Many of my experiences are with parents who are at the starting line of the grueling identification process and must come to grips with the diagnosis. As a classroom teacher of typical children with special education children mainstreamed into my classes, I have learned strategies to share with other teachers and parents. I am excited to pass along this information and some suggestions I wish someone would have given to me.

Shelli: When Patrick and I got married, I was determined to have a family and be a super mom. I knew it meant I would carry a heavy load, and I looked forward to that. I just had no idea it would mean doing this much. But I do it. I remember feeling overwhelmed and thinking I must just be a bad mother. Then I had a visit from a lady I now call my guardian angel, Elizabeth. She shared words of experience and wisdom that changed my life. Her support gave me the strength and encouragement to live my life and love it. Through this book, it is my hope to pass that knowledge on to others meeting the challenge of autism.

Elizabeth: When I was young, I just knew I would have a child with muscular dystrophy one day. My brother had it. I tested as a carrier. And I was okay with that. I loved my brother. He wasn't much different than other kids, except he couldn't walk. We could talk, he was incredibly smart, and sometimes, we fought. I had it all figured out. I was even glad this was my trial. What if I had a child with a mental disability? A child who couldn't communicate? Boy, I thought I was lucky.

I guess I am. I didn't have *a* child with *a* neurological communication disorder. I had three. And I consider myself the luckiest mother in the world. I am the mother of five passionately obsessive children. Three are diagnosed with autism. I have a degree in psychology that no one thought I would ever use. But I use it daily as I help my children discover they can do great things. I am an autism advocate and mother with powerful friends. I know how to get things done.

Finding the energy to actually do it is my lifelong pursuit. While looking for that energy, I have managed to speak to politicians, fund-raise, plan conferences, be on various boards serving autism families, write and blog, including an article in *Autism Asperger's Digest*.

If you ever thought, "It is not supposed to be this hard," then I hope in these pages, you will find wisdom to make good choices, comfort that you are not alone, and the strength to go on this incredible journey.

SECTION I

The Basics

If you don't ask the right questions, you don't get the right answers. A question asked in the right way often points to its own answer. Asking questions is the ABC of diagnosis. Only the inquiring mind solves problems.

—Edward Hodnett

Surviving the Diagnostic Process

Dr. B: Although some medical disorders may be diagnosed through blood tests or other procedures, autism is diagnosed by looking at the behavior of the child. This information may be gathered through direct observation by the medical professional or may be taken from information provided by the parent. The official diagnosis is normally given by a child psychiatrist, a developmental or behavioral pediatrician, or a pediatric neurologist. In some states a psychologist may give the official diagnosis. Children diagnosed with autism may fall anywhere along a full spectrum. Historically, autism spectrum disorder (ASD) included the diagnoses of classic autism, Asperger's syndrome, pervasive developmental disorder (PDD), Rhett's disorder, and childhood disintegrative disorder (CDD). Rhett's and CDD are rare. The DSM-5 (Diagnostic and Statistical Manual of Mental Disorders, Fifth Edition), is the 2013 update to the American Psychiatric Association's tool for classification and diagnosis. Currently the DSM-5 is undergoing change which will define all of these disorders as one inclusive diagnosis: autism spectrum disorder. Despite that change, a basic understanding of the different autism spectrum disorders will help you better understand your own child's needs and make it easier to communicate with the teachers, therapists, and medical professionals who are there to help your child. People previously diagnosed under the old classifications will retain their original diagnosis. Asperger's syndrome, although included in the diagnosis of ASD, will by most standards be set apart as having particular needs and therapeutic approaches. Additionally, the DSM-5 includes the diagnosis of social communication disorder, which includes difficulties with communication (verbal or nonverbal) without low cognitive ability.

Classic autism is characterized by deficits in both social interaction and communication. It includes hypersensitivity and hyposensitivity to stimuli from the environment.

Asperger's syndrome is recognized by the child's awkwardness in social interactions, but it does not impede his language skills.

Pervasive developmental disorder NOS (not otherwise specified) is a diagnosis given to a child who has some but not a significant number of characteristics of autism or who has relatively mild symptoms. PDD is often used synonymously with ASD or may be used as an umbrella term for the autism spectrum.

Childhood disintegrative disorder is rare condition in which children develop normally until at least two years of age but then demonstrate a severe loss of skills.

Rhett's disorder, also rare, is characterized by a loss of muscle tone. Rhett's is generally known to affect girls more than boys.

As a parent learning about your child's autism, you will hear many different terms including "high-functioning autism," "early learner," and "atypical autism." These terms can be confusing, not only because there are so many of them but also because they are used in different ways by various doctors, therapists, and other parents. Don't be shy about asking your treating professional to define terms he/she uses as we undergo this shift in terminology.

No matter what the doctors, teachers, or other parents label the disorder, your child's unique needs are your focus. No diagnostic label can tell you exactly what particular struggles or talents your child will have. Finding treatment that addresses your child's individual characteristics, rather than focusing on what label to attach, is the most helpful thing you can do for both your child and yourself. As it can possibly take years for a definitive diagnosis, proceed in your treatment plan with what you as the parent know about this child and his needs.

Elizabeth: As we offer an explanation of what autism is, we ask you to worry less about defining it and concentrate on a description of the traits that are manifesting themselves in your child. Also, be careful not to totally ignore those traits not presently showing in your child, because there is every possibility they may develop and will need to be addressed.

Dr. B: Beyond the official classification of autism spectrum disorder, you will be exposed at some point to a controversy involving the terminology used. There is a faction of parents and educators who are highly opposed to the term *autistic*, insisting instead on saying "child with autism." On the flip side of that is another group who is insulted by avoiding the term *autistic*. Their argument is that to avoid the term implies something is "wrong" with the child. You will be exposed to the term *Aspies*, which is a rather endearing reference to people with Asperger's. The term *Autists* is sometimes used, more in relation to adults with autism. Many times the reference will be simply to children with ASD (autism spectrum disorder).

A young lady named Michaela shared this story about her family's quest for answers to her brother's disabilities.

> My brother is twenty-two and was born before autism became what it is now. For the first six years of his life, my parents, sister, and I spent weekends traveling to specialists and pediatricians, attempting to determine why my little brother was nonverbal, shy, and had unusual reactions to pain and general external stimuli. The last specialist we visited completed a series of genetic tests to test for Fragile X and other disorders and finally diagnosed him as having pervasive developmental delay- not otherwise specified (PDD-NOS). There was never a mention of autism and my parents, both pharmacists, had never heard of the disorder. As my brother grew older and developed typical speech, his diagnosis then changed to "socially awkward." It was not until he was in high school, when a speech pathologist was working with him on his "face squeezing" tendencies, that ASD was mentioned.

Mrs. Nic: In your search for answers, you may run across some myths about children on the spectrum. In my private school, I worked with a little boy named Scotty who had been diagnosed with autism. He was nonverbal. His grandma would often bring him to school. She would say, "Oh, he will grow out of it." Scotty had a little sister, Jazzie, who started coming to my school with him the next year. I could see the grandma hoped Jazzie was going to be an example for Scotty. She would tell me when Scotty sees Jazzie doing things, he will "snap out of it." When the mom decided to have Jazzie evaluated for autism, it was hard for all the family. I think the grandma still had reservations about Jazzie's diagnosis because Jazzie said some words.

Mrs. Luck: I have worked with a significant number of families who also thought the child would someday "snap out of it." Although this gives the family hope, it is a false hope and places unfair burdens on the child. I knew a family of a low-functioning child who wanted their son's school to be teaching him at the fifth grade level so when he "snaps out of it," he won't be behind academically.

Dr. B: Other common myths are that all children with autism are geniuses or the reverse, that people with autism are all mentally challenged. The reality is the cognitive abilities of people with autism vary widely. Intelligence may lie anywhere on the range from very low to very high. One factor that fuels this misunderstanding is that children with autism tend to have "splinter skills." Their skills in various areas do not seem to all progress at the same speed. Some areas may lag behind while they are more advanced in other areas. Misunderstandings range from the statement we "can't help these kids" to "there is a genius hidden in each of them."

Demographics

D r. B: When I was taking special education courses in college, autism was considered to be rare. We were taught that the incidence was one child in 1,600. Now, a few decades later, the US Centers for Disease Control and Prevention gives the statistics at 1 in 50 students in the United States. Boys are being diagnosed five times more often than girls.[1] The Autism Society estimates 43,000 families will begin the autism journey this year.[2]

Autism crosses geographical, ethnic, social, and racial boundaries. According to the CDC, in the USA, rates are highest in Utah (1 in 47).[3] Globally, the rates in South Korea are said to top the charts (1 in 38).[4] There is some controversy about the study conducted in Korea, but it does highlight the fact that autism is a world-wide issue.

Elizabeth: My older son's autism is complicated by a rare chromosomal mutation that has resulted in brain damage, heart disease, and growth issues. His younger brother, who also has autism, is learning new skills every day as long as we are able to keep his seizures controlled.

After about a year of therapy in our home four days a week, Chase, the younger boy, had increased his compliance and loved his therapists. As each six weeks passed, we held our breath as he went through evaluations. Excited to chart his progression, I waited, expecting this to be the time, but it never came. The progression, the retention—it never came. It was all going in. It just didn't stick. He had not retained any skills.

Then came a second diagnosis, complex partial epilepsy. It had been misdiagnosed for years because only half of his brain seizes. Once he began anti-seizure medication, the seizures were controlled, and sleep came. Then seemingly overnight, he changed. Therapy was working. Things were beginning to stick. No longer were skills learned during the day and lost at night because sleep never came. Skills were now making their way to long-term memory instead of disappearing from short-term memory daily. His skill level skyrocketed within weeks.

Dr. B: Sometimes, the seizures start in early childhood, and other times, we don't see them appear until adolescence. In addition, children with autism are often reported to suffer immune system deficiencies. Allergies are prevalent. We also see a high number with severe sleep disturbances. Pica seems to be more common in children with autism than in the rest of the population. Pica is the desire to eat nonedible objects, such as dirt. This can lead to problems.

Causes—
Who is to Blame?

Dr. B: Autism was first introduced to mainstream America by Leo Kanner in 1943. He theorized autism was caused by a lack of warmth among the mothers and fathers of children who are affected.[5] This was the predominant theory for many years. The term "refrigerator mothers" was used to describe the relationship between the parents and the children. This stigma added a burden of guilt to parents already struggling with the challenges of raising a child with ASD. The theory of bad parenting as the cause of autism has since been ruled out by the scientific community. Although a variety of theories have followed Kanner's original theory, autism has no single, proven cause. There has been considerable debate about vaccines being a cause of autism.

Elizabeth: Jenny McCarthy, a quite public advocate of autism has referred to autism and the consequent recovery from symptoms as the equivalent of being hit by a bus. You may recover, but you will have always been hit by a bus. No matter how typical your behaviors and life may be, you will always have had autism.[6] Each time I think about the choice of vaccinating my children, I think of this metaphor. The difference is, I see the bus coming, and I have to decide if I should run like mad and push my child out of the way, or should I yell at them to duck and hope the bus passes safely over them. This is a choice no parent should ever have to make. I can assure you most parents who make the decision of whether or not to vaccinate in this generation do not do so lightly. We study, we research, and we pray. Then, we make a decision and live with it.

Dr. B: Studies have touted connections for a wide variety of causative factors, from living within a thousand feet of a freeway to parental age, infections, or brain abnormalities. There is simply no known single cause for autism. Current thought is that there may be many multiple factors contributing to the cause. Genetics, biological factors, and environment may all play a role.

Since the 1970s there has been evidence that there is a familial link to autism. Families who have one child with autism are at a higher recurrence risk than other families.[7] We do know autism is a complex syndrome. Researchers worldwide are searching for answers.

My caution to you is to not get too wrapped up in worrying about the cause or placing blame within your family. Some parents have told me their curiosity about the cause is based on them wanting to make an informed decision about having additional children. I can understand that. They feel more disposed to having additional pregnancies if the cause turned out to be something that would not be duplicated in subsequent children.

I sometimes feel like parents sitting in my office ask about the cause because they want to pinpoint which of them is to blame. In fact, some of them spontaneously confess to that as we chat. I see the icy stare of the mom as she wonders aloud if her son's autism is due to her husband smoking marijuana. I feel the chill in the air when the dad asks if this condition could have been caused by the mom not being responsive enough to a crying baby.

Scientists around the world are looking for answers to this complicated puzzle. That is their job. Our job is to direct our energy to help our children who show characteristics of being on the spectrum. If we want to promote autism research, there are plenty of opportunities to support those organizations with your time and resources. I urge you to become involved in those projects.

Prognosis

Elizabeth: In the diagnostic process, you may be told of your child's degree of severity. Don't let the diagnosis of "mildly autistic" or "requiring support" keep you from being diligent in your intervention efforts. If your child is diagnosed as "mild," I urge you not to simply accept your child's current state as "not that bad." Your child's autism will most likely not always be "mild." Without intervention, your child's autistic characteristics will probably worsen with age. An expanding and changing environment may cause him to withdraw or become more detached from reality.

Likewise, a diagnosis of "severe autism" or "requiring very substantial support" should not be seen as a deterrent to using your resources to the fullest extent possible to help your child. Help him become as successfully integrated into society as possible.

Use your child's diagnosis as a tool and starting place. A diagnosis is only the beginning, so don't let it be the end. A diagnosis is someone else's judgment of your child and is meant to help, not to discourage.

If you feel a diagnosis is incomplete or incorrect, please seek a second opinion. As a parent, trust your instincts. People do make mistakes, and autism can be puzzling, even to experts.

Be prepared that the diagnosis can be a lengthy process. If your child is extremely young (under or around two years old), an actual diagnosis may not be the most immediate goal. Don't wait for the final diagnosis before you begin your intervention process. However, if the lack of an official diagnosis is keeping your child from receiving the help he needs, you should push for a diagnosis as soon as possible.

During the testing process, you will be given questions to answer. Don't try to hide anything, thinking it doesn't matter or it is normal. A team of professionals will pore over this information. Let them decide the importance of a certain behavior. Please make a copy of this before you turn it in. Keep your responses and your test results in a personal file. If you ever need them in the future for any reason, you will already have them on hand.

When our daughter was diagnosed at thirty months of age, the team we were working with said they were afraid to tell us. They kept trying to protect us with gentle words. They were quite pleasantly surprised at our acceptance of Nicole's diagnosis. We basically took a deep breath and said, "Okay, so what do we do?" We now had a starting point and knew which direction to head. Not knowing what was wrong had been torture to us. With this new information, we could begin helping her.

Dr. B: Although there are multiple theories about the cause of autism, there is widespread agreement about one thing—the importance of early intervention. According to the Autism Society, early diagnosis and intervention are critical in improving a child's behavior and functioning. Without early intervention, the symptoms of autism can worsen. This could result in symptoms becoming more severe and may create the added burden of increased life time costs. [8]

SECTION II

Red Flags

If all my possessions were taken away from me with one exception, I would choose to keep the power of communication, for by it I would soon regain all the rest.

—Daniel Webster

Communication

Dr. B: There is a saying widely heard in the autism community. It states, "If you met a person with autism, you met one person with autism."[9] The point of this bit of wisdom is that while many people may be on the autism spectrum, each one is vastly different from the next. Like a million snowflakes, there are commonalities that identify each of them as a member of this group, but they differ so much from one another that it can be misleading to rely totally on generalizations. Skills, intelligence, and personality traits can vary widely. However, there is a set of characteristics that many people on the spectrum share, as compared to their age-matched peers. These are commonly referred to as red flags or indicators of the presence of ASD. Each person may have any number of these characteristics, and in varying degrees. Although a child on the spectrum may not have all of these characteristics, each of these traits seems to be quite prevalent, although not universal, among the children in this population.

Elizabeth: The interesting thing about red flags is that as parents, we often misinterpret them as strengths, gifts, and intense personalities. We watch our child lining up toys in rows and see a child with advanced organizational skills. Our child who obsesses over moving parts and is more interested in how a toy works than how to play with it is branded an engineer by fourteen months. We see a very brave child who seems to have no fear and a very strong child because he doesn't react to pain. As a new parent, we look at our beautiful child, unaware that there are studies that link innocence and beauty with lack of emotional expression. We notice they like to be by themselves and congratulate ourselves on what a good job we have done raising a confident and independent child. And oh, can they memorize! Are there many toddlers who can repeat lines from the *Lion King* and *Phantom of the Opera* nonstop? But as the intensity and rate of these behaviors increase, it isn't cute anymore. We realize these endearing qualities we valued are all red flags of developmental problems. They are red flags of autism. So what was once memorizing skills is now echolalia and holds no conversational value. It is important to know the red flags for yourselves and for others.

Shelli: Joshuah was my first child. I watched every move he made. His fascination with rocks was intoxicating to me. He was almost two. He was saying *hi, bye-bye, outside,* and a number of other words. But now, he was quiet and just wanted to be left alone. I would try to get his attention. He wouldn't look at me. I was not thinking something was wrong with this beautiful little boy. I thought he was just going to be a quiet, strong-willed child, with his own way of doing things. We would struggle to take him anywhere. He would scream and make a scene in restaurants and grocery stores. We noticed he was a little more calm when we would pack some match box cars, a Sippy cup, and his light-blue blanket. I was just randomly talking to our pediatrician about some of these things at a well-baby checkup, and she looked at me and said, "Shelli, do you think he has autism?"

I gave her a quick response, "No." But I left the office and started thinking, "Does my son have something going on with him?" I had been given lots of parenting advice up to this point and had just thought I was not a very good mom.

I was already pregnant with my second child and made my mind up this was my last one. Joshuah was going on two and would not sleep. I would rearrange his room, and it would seem to throw him all off. His sleep patterns would be disturbed for weeks. The couple of times we went out of town, he would not sleep the entire time we were gone. It was exhausting. Everything had to be just so-so with him. I thought it was amazing seeing his well-sorted Fruit Loops on his high chair tray. All the signs were adding up. I was ready. Let's just see what the doctor says about Joshuah having autism. I took the doctor my list of things we were seeing in my son. It didn't take her long. She reached over and grabbed me a box of tissues and said, "Shelli, your son has autism." She referred us to a neurologist. She said she could not give us an official diagnosis, but the neurologist could.

Two months later, we got in to see the neurologist. We had a questionnaire we had to answer. We went in with mixed feelings. Maybe he would not see autism; maybe my son was just hyperactive and stubborn. During our visit, Josh was holding flash cards on the wall and watching them fall to the ground, repeatedly. He didn't even look up when the doctor called out as he came through the door. After thousands of questions, we were done. Joshuah fit the criteria for a diagnosis of autism. The doctor told us there was not a cure for autism, but therapy would help give us a better outcome. We left the doctor's office feeling very heavy. My husband and I were pretty quiet as we left that appointment. We had so much information to sift through. The doctor handed us a stack of papers with information about autism. Now that we knew the difficulties we were having with our son were normal for a kid suffering with autism and this was not a product of bad parenting, I felt some kind of relief and a new form of stress all at once.

We got Joshuah plugged into First Steps, a state-sponsored program for children birth to age three. This program was amazing. Everyone was telling me early intervention was the key, and this program provided just that. They came to my home, which was a nice feature of the program, and provided services such as occupational therapy for sensory integration and speech-language therapy. The teachers modeled the use of applied behavior analysis (ABA therapy), which is behavior modification. The service coordinator warned me about ABA being really intense. They came to my home four days a week for an hour and a half. I wanted it. I had heard really positive things about ABA therapy. Having strangers come into my home was stressful at first, but the staff just quickly became part of our family. They didn't care that

I had messes or that I looked exhausted from no sleep; they were there to help. I loved every one of them dearly.

Dr. B: Parents tell me they were happy and proud that their infant was so "good." Their babies seem content, seldom crying out for attention or to have their needs met. It's interesting that some parents tell of resisting the diagnosis when professionals or other parents suggest autism, yet others go to the doctor armed with the list of red flags they are seeing, only to be told the child will "grow out of it" or "kids all grow at their own rate." When parents share their histories with me, they often say the mom had the first clue. Dads might either trust the mom and go along with her instincts or may remain resistant to the diagnosis for years. Parents have told me, "I think I always knew, from day one, that he was different, but I didn't know what it was."

Mrs. Nic: Tony is a typically developing eight-year-old that has a brother diagnosed with autism. Tony explained to me that "some people have a little touch of autism, and other people get it pretty bad, and my brother has kind of an in-between amount of it."

Shelli: Having two children on the spectrum is a lot of fun sometimes. I am like most parents that have multiple children. I get to observe on a day-to-day basis how autism has affected them in different ways. Each child is so unique. Both kids have their special personality traits that make up who they are. Autism doesn't define who they are—it just plays a part in how they individually react to their environment. This is really why it is so important when working with these kids that we focus on a child as a person, not just "this is someone with autism." For example, my older child hates to be in a room with three or more people. It makes him really nervous, and he has a major meltdown. He will do whatever it takes to get out. He will try to grab my hand and do his best to lead me to the door. My younger child gets excited when she gets in a room with people. She loses all control. It is like an adrenaline rush for her. She starts laughing out loud, flapping her hands, and spinning in circles. While my son throws himself on the floor and screams, she is delighted.

Dr. B: One of the most heartbreaking aspects of autism is that it sometimes robs children of skills they have previously acquired. Children who are on target for developmental milestones suddenly regress and lose skills they have mastered. Although some doctors give this a different diagnosis, for educational purposes, it often falls into the autism spectrum. Parents have described to me feeling their child was "stolen" from them at this point. One likened it to having your child kidnapped from your arms as you stand by helplessly. Children with ASD are at an increased risk of seizures or other medical issues that may affect the continuum of development.

Elizabeth: When Nicole was diagnosed, we did everything we could. We were told to do it, and we did. It wasn't easy, but she was learning. Behaviors were improving. We were nine months into the interventions, and there was no stopping her. Then one morning, things seemed to go backward. I decided to give it a week before panicking. I forced myself every day to think she was just having a bad day, but it was gone. Everything she had learned just seemed to disappear. We were at square one.

Her team at school held my hand and assured me this is often the natural course of autism. They told me children who suffer with autism often cycle, gaining skills and apparently losing them. They encouraged me to hang in there, that hope was not lost. I learned that children who suffer regression rarely regress back to where they started and relearning those lost skills will come faster each time around. They were right.

So the question is, "Is this complication related to the autism, or is it a learning process?" There is some question about if this process is a built-in mechanism to solidify skills learned and increase long-term retention or just another part of autism.

There are times when regression sticks. While it is heartbreaking, it is not the end of learning. It may indicate there is something else going on that needs attention, even medical attention or intervention. To work through regression, you may need to work with your child in new and different ways. New techniques may stimulate neuro-pathways not previously tapped into. Mix it up and try again. Never give up.

Nathan's recovery from regression has come slowly, but just when we make adjustments in his life for those lost skills, he gives us a peek into his mind and capabilities. After only a handful of words in months, out will pop a perfectly articulate sentence that is not due to echolalia but rather a well thought out purposeful message. While his reading is gone, letters and their sounds remain. And hope abounds.

Dr. B: Humans are by nature social animals. One of the most severe punishments we give to prisoners is to put them in isolation, eliminating all opportunity for communication with others. Teenagers who misbehave often have their social communication cut off as a consequence—the phone, the texting, and the e-mail. Communication is our most basic connection to others in our world. It allows us to share ideas, express feelings, and ask questions. To eliminate the ability to communicate effectively interferes with those essential interactions. Children who display autistic characteristics by definition struggle with various aspects of communication skills. In order to succeed in communicating with others, it is essential to develop a functional use of language.

Speech disorder, or the inability to say words clearly, is not a defined part of autism, but it often is seen in children with autism. The way we pronounce words is referred to as articulation. Childhood apraxia of speech is a severe motor speech disorder that is believed by many to occur in a higher percentage of children on the autism spectrum than in the general population. Such a severe speech disorder may make it even more difficult for children with autism to learn to communicate effectively. On the other hand, children with autism that may display mild speech problems are often overlooked for remediation because in the grand scheme of the child's challenges, a lisp just doesn't seem so important.

Mrs. Nic: Inability to say certain speech sounds can drastically change the meaning of what the child is trying to convey. We were taking our integrated kindergarten class to visit a farm. In preparation for the visit, we discussed the various animals we would see. Most of the children knew we get eggs from a chicken. When I asked them what we get from a cow, Jaden volunteered what sounded like *cow semen*. It took me a minute to figure out he was trying to say *calcium*.

Dr. B: The speech we produce also has various vocal characteristics. Voice disorders can take many forms. Any aberration that calls attention to itself, or does not sound like the voice of an age and sex matched peer, is considered to be abnormal. This includes voices that are of poor quality, problems with volume, and problems in pitch. These abnormalities are often noted as early as the babbling stage in the infant.

The quality of a voice may be distorted if it sounds perpetually hoarse, harsh, or breathy. He may sound too nasal or not nasal enough. These voice disorders may or may not have a true medical basis. Medical problems would need to be ruled out before a speech-language pathologist could intervene.

Problems in volume may be heard as a voice that is routinely too loud or too soft. Some children with autism prefer to whisper and need to be taught to speak in a typical volume in order to make their wants and needs known. Others tend to shout and must learn to moderate their volume for an "inside voice."

Children who speak in a flat intonation, or a monotone, are said to have problems in pitch. The voice is compared against persons of the same age and sex. A vocal pitch that does not match that expectation would call attention to the speaker, and therefore would be considered a disorder. Some young boys with autism speak in a high pitch commonly known as a falsetto. As they mature into adulthood, this falsetto voice becomes socially unacceptable. We normally try to help the child minimize any characteristics that make him seem different from other children.

Language impairment is a core symptom of autism. Children with ASD have a difficult time understanding spoken language. Known as receptive language, this is an area of development that can be very difficult for a child with autism. Academic success depends upon the ability to understand the spoken word. Being able to follow directions is a critical skill for a child to be successful in school or in the family structure. In order for communication to have an element of reciprocity with others, receptive language is essential. Many speech-language pathologists find it helpful to focus on understanding before production. A child who displays verbal language that is meaningless does not actually have functional expressive language.

Mrs. Luck: As children on all points of the spectrum are very literal, be sure you are saying what you think you are saying if you expect them to understand you. I had a veteran third-grade teacher very upset with a student. "He is defiant, he challenges me in the classroom, and I won't have it. Do something about it! I tell the class, 'Put your books up', and he just sits there with his books on his desk. I tell him again, and he picks them up but does not put them away." I asked the teacher, "Exactly what do you want him to do?" She replied, "Put his books on the shelf *under* his seat." I advised, "Then, tell him that." The student was no longer defiant when the teacher wanted the desk cleared off now that it was clear she wanted the books put *down*, not *up*.

To make your communication with an ASD person easier, avoid using words like, *everyone*, *no one*, *all*, *none*, *always*, or *never*. Sentences such as "Everyone likes ice cream" or "No one likes to walk to school in the rain" will likely result in an argument you cannot win. While a typically developing child will accept a sentence such as "Never run in the hall," an autistic child may give you quite an argument, listing situations when it might be appropriate.

Jason had been in trouble in his class. The problem was quickly escalating, and he referred to the teacher as a liar. When I did a drill down on the problem, he was outraged because the teacher had accused him of "talking all through the class" and had said to him, "You *never* listen." He correctly stated that while he did talk a lot, it was certainly not *all* through the class, and he *did* listen sometimes. He felt wrongly accused because of the descriptive words she used.

Dr. B: Greg was upset after hearing the TV commercial for baked goods by Sara Lee. Their slogan claims, "Nobody doesn't like Sara Lee." Each day, when I saw Greg, he reminded me of the commercial's claim along with the fact that his cousin doesn't like cake, so therefore the commercial isn't true. He was indignant that they make such misleading claims and was relentless in chastising them for what he felt was an ill-advised jingle.

Mrs. Luck: When you are communicating with people on the spectrum, avoid making promises or statements that can be perceived as a promise. If a situation ever comes along that forces a change in what you have promised, the ASD person's world may be bounced into turmoil, and he may not be easily redirected. The first week of school a new student, Ryan, was mildly but persistently misbehaving and the teacher told him emphatically that she was going to "call your mom and dad to discuss this disruptive behavior." He escalated into a major violent behavior episode, yelling profanities, kicking chairs, punching walls, and screaming, "My dad is in prison, and you can't call him, and you said you are going to, and you can't, so you are a —— liar."

Mrs. Nic: Their world is defined by this concrete, literal thought pattern. Jake came into class and had a bloodied knee, obviously the result of a fall. I asked him if he fell down, and he told me he had. In an effort to find out if he had fallen on the playground, in the parking lot, etc., I asked him, "Where did you fall?" He looked at me like I was crazy and answered matter-of-factly, "On the ground." *Of course,* I thought. "Good answer, Jake." I knew Jake was wondering why I would ask such a silly question with such an obvious answer.

Dr. B: One day, the seven-year-old boys in Ms. Susan's class were doing a particularly great job on a language project. She was so proud of their accomplishments, she excitedly told them, "Great job! You guys are on fire today!" Will started screaming and running, thinking that he was really on fire, really burning. Ms. Susan had her hands full, trying to calm him down and convince him he was not *actually* on fire. When I saw Will about six months later, he proudly told me, "I'm on fire today. That doesn't really mean I'm on fire. It means I am doing good work."

A person who has Asperger's syndrome often has mastered the mechanics of language but lacks the pragmatic skills, otherwise known as the social aspects of language. He may have an exceptional vocabulary but have little knowledge of how to use language socially. The child may have poor conversational skills, including either the inability to initiate a conversation or the inability to maintain or follow the conversation. He may not know how to socially greet others or to shift his conversational style to match different social settings. Most adults have learned to develop several sets of language skills and social skills. The way you talk to your boss is different from the way you talk to your children. This is known as using different social registers. Children on the spectrum may have only one set of pragmatic skills or social rules. These children appear to be rude or aloof because of this. They can take the school rules and apply them to the home setting and sound like the little professor, or using home rules, tell the teacher he needs "to go poop." Pragmatics is just one of the areas of language that may be deficient.

Other children may show difficulties in syntax or the grammar of our language. Each language on earth is governed by its unique set of rules. We commonly know these rules as *grammar*. Children with poor syntactical skills construct awkward sentences. When they are very young, children actually follow "children's rules" ("me want a cookie"), but as they mature, their grammatical structures typically evolve into adult rules. A child with low syntactical skills may generate a sentence that is less complex than the speech of his age-matched peers, or he may consistently form grammatically incorrect sentences.

The third common symptom of language disorders involves problems of semantics or meaning of the language. These children may have limited vocabulary or may have word retrieval issues. In addition, the child may tend to overuse words that lack specificity, such as *thing* or *stuff*. He may often select a wrong word, as he has difficulty recalling the word he wants to say. Understanding the meaning of the words in the language we use is crucial for a child if we expect him to make language useful to himself. He needs to learn, for example, that *jump* means something different than *jumped*, and *jumping* is yet another concept. He needs to learn a boy is referred to as *he* while *she* refers to a girl. He will need to understand *cat* refers to one cat while *cats* refers to multiple cats. Small changes in the construction of a word might totally change the meaning of the word. This is very difficult for some students. Pronouns are a particularly difficult concept for our children with autism to understand. Their echolalia seems to be to blame for part of that confusion. When I go into Mr. Dave's class during snack time and ask, "Do you want more?" five little voices answer back, "You want more!" as they hold out their hands in anticipation.

Mrs. Luck: When working with Jason, I say, "My name is Mrs. Luck. What is *your* name?" His likely answer is "*Your* name is Jason." It has also been suggested that some of the pronoun confusion relates to a lack of awareness of *self*.

Other times the pronoun confusion is not related to the echolalia. When I told Tim his shoe was untied, he answered, "Oh, he is? Okay, I'll fix him." When I asked Aiden where his cookie was, he said, "I ate her."

Dr. B: Children may show delays or disorders in either the ability to understand language or to actually generate it. The issues described above (syntax, semantics, or pragmatics) might each be manifested in the child's receptive (understanding) or expressive (producing) language skills, or a combination of both. Parents tell me, "He understands everything we say to him, yet he doesn't talk at all." On the opposite side of the coin, some children seem extremely verbal and talk very well, yet they really struggle to understand what others are saying to them.

Elizabeth: One thing about a child on the spectrum is that when his language is delayed or lacking, he may have no means to compensate. He might use some broad gestures to fill his needs, such as leading you by the hand to the refrigerator to receive a drink, but that broad gesturing is pretty limited. If you can help him refine those gestures by teaching him how to use another form of communication, doors will begin to open, especially refrigerator doors. Nicole was an avid signer. She would give the signs for "cookie" and "please" over and over. The sign for "please" is making a little circle on your chest. Nicole would take her little palm and rub it slow and hard in that circle. I usually gave in. She was just so cute.

Dr. B: You may hear language described as either *delayed* or *disordered*. These terms may be used by either the medical or the educational professionals. One way to understand the difference between these two issues is to visualize a class of children all in a single file line. Imagine they are all going to walk to the playground. Now think about the possibility of two children walking more slowly than the others and getting far behind. They will eventually reach the playground, following the same path as the others, but they will be delayed reaching the goal. Now imagine two of the students go off the planned path and take a wrong turn. They head off in their own direction, not following the others. Their journey can now be described as disordered. Without intervention, they will likely not end up where they need to be.

Classroom teachers are not trained to be highly skilled in language therapy. While they are experts in teaching the progression of language skills to the typically developing child, they need more help in teaching the child with special needs. Some of them will embrace that support while others have admitted resenting the extra work placed on them.

Language is commonly thought of as being expressed verbally. This is not always the case. Language may be written language or sign language of different methods. Language might even be expressed by the use of pictures or communication devices. These alternative methods have proven to be helpful with many nonverbal children. You will often find the most effective forms of these systems are modifications of a more formal program. In 1994, Lori Frost, a speech-language pathologist, teamed with Dr. Andy Bondy, an educator, to develop a system using small pictures that a child could exchange for a wanted item or action ("Picture Exchange Communication System").[10] This is known as a picture exchange communication system or PECS. This intervention provides a method for the child to make his functional wants and needs known to others in his environment by handing the listener a small picture. The association of each picture to the desired item must be taught to the child. Once mastered, the system can be used in the home, school, and community. Many successful programs actually use some modified form of the original PECS, adjusting the program to an individual child's needs.

Shelli: My children's behaviors have changed so much with age and their increased abilities to communicate. Joshuah opened up to new things when he was introduced to PECS. It was easier to tell him what we expected of him.

Dr. B: Using a form of sign language is also helpful with some non-verbal children. As with the PECS, the individualized education program often includes a modified version of a manual sign, making it easier for the child to master. The terms *total communication* or *simultaneous communication* refer to programs that use verbal speech concurrently with a nonverbal method. Many parents and therapists feel a simultaneous method is the most effective.

As our society becomes more and more tech-savvy, the field of augmentative assistive devices for speech and language has increased. There is a large variety of AACs now available depending on the cognitive level of the student and the budget of the family. The iPad is quickly gaining popularity with therapists and families as an electronic assistance to communication. There are commercial apps available that give the student a means of expressing his needs. Most children seem to enjoy the use of the technology. Parents often worry that by promoting the use of nonverbal means of communication, they will be reducing the chances of the child ever producing meaningful verbal language. However, just the opposite appears to be true. Studies report that aided approaches and sign language actually have the potential to enhance and quicken the development of spoken language in children on the spectrum.

Mrs. Nic: I suggest parents who invest in the iPad (or any similar device) as an augmentative means of communication purchase a really good protective rubber cover for it. Electronic devices are expensive and need to be protected from accidents. Small hands are often clumsy, and children sometimes show poor judgment in caring for expensive items. Another suggestion I have heard from parents is if you intend to use the iPad as a communication device, do *not* allow the child to use it for games. Get some other system for the child to play games on, but keep the iPad as a communication tool, if that is your intention. To allow games to be played on the device you choose as your alternative communication device will be distracting to the child, confusing, and will likely result in child-parent conflict. I knew a parent who stayed religiously with this rule and, then one day allowed the games "just this once." She regretted that moment of weakness for months to come. To keep peace in the family, keep the uses of the various electronic devices separate.

Mrs. Luck: Communication difficulties not only include being very literal, but also problems in understanding inferences, rhetorical questions, multiple meaning words, or body language among other things. The social aspect of language eludes them and must be taught.

Dr. B: The most rapid and intense period of the development of speech and language is commonly acknowledged to occur during the first three years of a child's life. This is a period when the brain is developing and maturing in many areas. A child's early skills appear to develop best in a highly stimulating world, full of rich sounds, interesting sights, and reinforcing exposure to the speech and language of others. These stimuli produce the desire to interact with those around him. One of the earliest forms of infant communication is when the baby learns that a cry will bring food and comfort. From an amazingly early age, neonates can recognize the sound of their mothers' or fathers' voices.

Soon, the infant is able to make different oral sounds and begins to enjoy the attention this brings to him. As he gains more control over the speech mechanism, he becomes more proficient in producing the sounds he hears others making. Typically, by the age of six months, the baby is making repetitive sounds, such as *dada* or *baba*. Children who do not babble by the age of twelve months may be exhibiting signs of either autism or other developmental delays.

Early in a typical baby's development, he learns to delight in a social reciprocity using gestures. Waving bye-bye is an example of the child learning to socially enjoy a back-and-forth communication with another person. Lack of early gesturing, or the disappearance of that skill, may be considered to be a red flag. Similarly, the same pattern in speech skills allows the child to communicate or interact with his world and, in turn, form a base for the development of communication skills.

Mrs. Nic: If the child has begun babbling, waving bye-bye, throwing kisses, and playing pat-a-cake, then can no longer do those sounds and gestures, the parent should seek out answers for the child's loss of skills.

Elizabeth: Overall, they just have a really hard time interacting with others. It seems like they would rather just be left alone and are withdrawn. They fail to reciprocate both socially and emotionally.

Dr. B: Children diagnosed as being on the spectrum often show inconsistent responses to people and things. A toddler may turn to the sound of his name at one point but may not react the next time. The inconsistency of his responses may be unnerving to the parent. At this point, some parents make an appointment to get the child's hearing checked to rule out a hearing problem. He may show you good eye contact one day, then no eye contact for the next week. There is just no pattern to the responses. Even more unnerving is that he may totally ignore something one day, such as a certain sound, but then get extremely upset by the same sound the next time he is exposed to it. One day, he may seem to not even notice the door bell, but the next day, he may cover his ears and scream as though the noise causes true pain.

Elizabeth: You may notice an inappropriate response to a sound or no response at all. Hearing can be seen as hyper and hypo in the same child. Your child may seek out extremely loud noises because of the overwhelming attraction to this stimulus. He may run toward a fire alarm rather than running away. This same child may not be able to tolerate the sound of running water. Children with autism are often seen covering their ears. Nathan covers his ears whenever there is a change in volume, especially in vocal stimulation. Unless your child shows signs of distress, he is probably not in any pain. A child with autism will sometimes make noises (often loud) to act as a filter to the constant irritation in hearing too much extraneous noise.

I had Nicole at a parade one Saturday with her cousins. Children began to crowd around us as candy was thrown. Before I realized it, Nicole was gone. It happened so fast, I could still feel her hand in mine. But I saw a man jump from the crowd and grab my child as she walked right in front of a fire engine whose sirens were blaring. All the while, she was staring blankly at this truck. I was horrified.

A child with auditory sensitivities will sometimes resort to hiding under tables and chairs in large rooms full of noisy children. Desensitizing your child to these irritants is a step-by-step process. Learning to recognize these sensitivities will help your child avoid overloads that cause a breakdown in behavior.

Mrs. Nic: We worked with a preteen named Adam who would quietly sob sometimes when music would play. Other times, he would happily dance or sing along laughing when the same song played. One day, we took the class to the movie theater to see a Disney movie. When the music started, he stood up proudly and happily made movements of an orchestra conductor, with tears rolling down his cheeks.

Dr. B: Echolalia is the repetition of what someone else has said. It is a normal part of learning speech and language for a typically developing child. Children with autism tend to display echolalia more frequently, and it lasts for a longer time than with the typical child. Some parents have stated they feel echolalia to be the most common way their child's communication differs from the verbal behavior of age-matched peers. The words the child repeats after hearing them from someone else may or may not have communicative intent. An example of this happened in a social skills class. The topic was *family*, and each child was telling what his dad does. James said, "My dad is a carpenter." Jack said, "My dad is a fire fighter." When it was Darren's turn, he announced to the class, "My dad is a douche!"

Mrs. Nic: Josie is ten years old, and this year, she repeats the word "*shazamm*" continually all day. As far as we can tell, there is no meaning to the word, just a word she repeats.

Mrs. Luck: Jonas was twelve when he came to our school. He repeated the phrase "two weeks" all day long for months—well, actually for the three years I knew him.

Shelli: Both of my kids are functionally nonverbal, although my daughter's vocabulary is growing. She does communicate by echolalia. This is a lot of fun for me at times. She repeats movies, songs, just random things she has heard. She will say phrases in the same pitch and tone it was said in. She will be in public and hear a child crying, which she thinks is funny and entertaining, and she will echo what she is hearing, often at very inconvenient times.

Dr. B: When a phrase is repeated incessantly, I liken it to when a typical person has a song "stuck in your head." That happens to all of us, but normally, we are able to shake it off in a relatively short time. These *earworms* invade the speech of the child with autism and become a trademark sound he produces for a given amount of time.

Echolalia may be immediate or may be delayed. Delayed echolalia might be relevant to the situation or might be totally random to what is happening around him. In some cases, it might be situational, triggered by what is happening at the moment. Many children with autism decrease their use of echolalia as they master more functional language skills. In other cases, we see echolalia increase when a child is in a stressful situation. Sometimes, the echolalia seems to serve a purpose for the child. In conversational turn taking, he may realize it is his "turn" to contribute to the conversation but not know what to say. He cannot generate a response, so he pulls something from his repertoire.

Mrs. Luck: Here is an example of kids who want to join in the conversation but don't know what to say or just simply lack the language skills to interact. The kids in the self-contained room were very excited about going to a movie in the cafeteria.

"We get to see a movie."

"And we are going to get popcorn."

"And we are going to get pop."

"And it's going to be fun."

Our guy who is on the spectrum added, "And the dish ran away with the spoon."

Another example was when a new volunteer named Mr. John was helping put together a swing set at our special education day service center. I sent Michael, one of the adult clients, out to help him. Mr. John, who has a degree in engineering, laid out all the parts of the swing set on the grass. Michael walked around and around the pieces and, looking down at them, said, "That's the top."

Mr. John said, "Okay" and moved all the pieces around to the direction Michael indicated. Michael walked around the pieces again, stopped on the other side, and announced, "That's the top."

Mr. John was a little ticked, said, "Okay," and moved all the pieces again. After about the fourth time, Mr. John turned to Michael and said, "You're really not much help" to which Michael looked at him blankly and said, "That's the top." Maybe we should have warned Mr. John that Michael says, "That's the top" every few minutes all day long. This is an example of how saying words is not the same thing as having language.

Dr. B: Some children rely on echolalia as a method to attempt to answer a question. I asked six-year-old Anna, "Do you want to paint?" She answered, "Do you want to paint." The next day, when I again came into the classroom, she saw I had painting supplies in my hands, she reached for the supplies and said, "Do you want to paint!"

Echolalia may extend to a characteristic known as scripting. Scripting goes hand-in-hand with echolalia. Many children with autism can recite long segments from a movie they have watched or even a conversation they have heard. Some parents feel scripting is proof of their child's intelligence.

Elizabeth: Scripting is something that is recognized as interfering with typical social norms. Therapies often use *extinguishing* as a target goal for scripting. Scripting never really bothered me as a parent. I actually attribute it to Nicole's incredible ability to memorize scripts and act. For me, worrying about what other people think as my children continuously recite *Green Eggs and Ham* while recounting the events of the day is something I don't normally waste my energy on. But there is more to it. A child who is verbally replaying events, movies, or schedules continuously loses the ability to focus. Their minds and mouths are so full that what they should be learning doesn't stand a chance. There is no room for vital input if your child is constantly scripting. Also, if they use scripting as a coping mechanism, their real needs are not being addressed and productive coping strategies are not being developed.

I think there is often a fine line between scripting and practicing. As we guide our children, we need to look at what is being accomplished by it. Does it serve a purpose for our child? If our child continues to script, we also need to look at the social implications. We all hope our children will hold jobs one day, and scripting could cause issues in the workplace. As with all therapies and strategies, we must not forget who we are doing this for. Extinguishing scripting must be for the benefit of your child and take its proper place in the prioritizing of skills needing to be developed.

The importance of communication is felt in every aspect of a child's life. Children who cannot use language might show frustration and resort to maladaptive behaviors. The abilities to make friends, to maintain friendships, to succeed in school, and to fully participate in life are all founded on communication. When children can use language in some form to make their wants and needs known, their world becomes a much friendlier place. Almost every topic of discussion on how to help our children revolves around a core need for communication skills.

Sensory Issues

Dr. B: In some modern cultures, it is a sign of disrespect for a speaker to engage in eye contact with his listener. Unfortunately for American children diagnosed with ASD, this is not the case in the USA. People engaged in conversation are expected to establish eye contact with one another. Our social convention leads us to believe people who avoid eye contact while in a conversation may be *shifty* or have something to hide. Young adults with ASD who have higher level language skills have explained their aversion to eye contact. They say it is like "seeing a hundred dizzying snapshots of the face in a minute" as they look at the speaker. That, coupled with a struggle to even recognize the face, is disturbing to the person with autism.

Facial recognition is a challenge to many on the spectrum. One parent described to me how her son would go around the house methodically turning over family photos so as to avoid seeing the faces. He would even turn small figurines and knick-knacks around to make the little faces point toward the wall. Although eye contact can be taught and many can overcome this ally debilitating characteristic, it often requires constant reminders by those around him. You will notice some children who have poor or inconsistent eye contact but use "gaze checks" to briefly give fleeting eye contact to the speaker repeatedly through the conversation. Some have associated this with the fact that they often do not look straight on at objects at all, whether human or nonhuman, but rather use their peripheral vision.

A teacher I worked with, Ms. DeeDee, has Asperger's syndrome. She told me she has taught herself a trick of looking "near the eyes." She said not only does she hate looking in another person's eyes, she actually feels violated when someone looks directly into her eyes. She explained it feels like someone has invaded her privacy and looked into her soul. She is simply following the golden rule: do unto others as you would have them do unto you. She does not want others looking into her eyes, so she will not violate you by looking into yours. She feels that she is doing the other person a favor by avoiding eye contact.

Elizabeth: Probably the most acclaimed red flag is lack of eye contact. This is the first question we are asked: "Does your child make eye contact with you?" Often, before we seek professional help, the answer is yes. Then it is explained that a fleeting glance is not eye contact. It must be a sustained gaze. "Does my child do that?" we ask ourselves. Sometimes, the answer is no. "No, he doesn't make eye contact."

Mrs. Luck: Eye contact is often a struggle, requiring a delicate balance. Be careful not to overemphasize the importance of having the student look you in the eyes.

I had a fifth grade student who had been drilled by his parents to "look 'em in the eye, son." This little guy would lock eyes with me as he walked into the room and never break eye contact the entire hour of speech. It was a little unnerving. I had to teach him to look toward me but not stare.

Because they avoid eye contact, kids with autism do not see the world the same way as others do. I saw one of my former students in the hall at the beginning of the school year. For several days, he passed by my door, never speaking to me. Then one day, as he passed, he smiled and said, "Mrs. Luck, I didn't know it was you until I saw your flip-flops."

Our principal and assistant principals dressed for Halloween as the Cat in the Hat and Thing 1 and Thing 2. They had body costumes on but wore no masks and had no makeup. Their faces were clearly visible. One of my kids said, "That's the principal and his two assistants. I recognized their hair."

Mrs. Nic: One day, we were conducting a social skills class made up of children with a variety of challenges. The counselor, who had been working with this class all year, had a bad case of laryngitis that day, causing her voice to be hoarse and raspy. She explained her voice problem to the class. Seven-year-old Evan came into class late, sat in the front row, and as the teacher spoke, he was clearly agitated. He raised his hand and said, "I can't figure out who you are because your voice doesn't sound right! Are you Ms. Jeannie or Ms. Bowen? I can't hear who you are." Although he settled down when she explained why her voice sounded unidentifiable to him, it would never have been an option for him to simply *look* at her face and see who was speaking.

Shelli: Visual perception is interesting when talking about autism. It is so hard for these kids to focus on specific details when their minds are taking snapshots of everything around them in milliseconds. I believe when you ask for eye contact you are helping them pull their focus in more clearly. I can also see that this is why it is hard for many ASD individuals to read facial clues.

I sometimes think eye contact is about trust. I think the kid has a harder time with eye contact with unfamiliar people than he would otherwise. I think it is easier for ASD kids to make eye contact with people who stop and take time to build a relationship (trust) with them. It is such an important part of communication that I really feel like eye contact should be one of the first goals taught. I have heard from verbal people on the spectrum that it actually hurts to make eye contact.

Mrs. Luck: One day, as I was working with seven-year-old James, he noticed someone walk past the window. It was a staff member who was very familiar to him. The staff member happened to be wearing a green shirt. The movement of the person passing the window caught James's eye, and he asked me, "Where is that green shirt going?" Although he had known that teacher for two years, he automatically relied on cues other than facial recognition to identify the person.

Mrs. Nic: I knew a teenager named Jason who explained that he could not both listen and look at the speaker's face at the same time. When teachers insisted he look at them as they talk, he could not follow the lecture because it was so disturbing to watch the speaker's face. The teachers felt he was disrespectful in class because he either closed his eyes or looked at the ceiling in order to follow the lecture. At the parent-teacher meeting, Jason's mom asked the complaining history teacher, "Would you rather have him look at you while you lecture and not be able hear a word you say or look away so he can understand what you are saying?" Jason's mom also gave us a great tip. A neurologist suggested to her that when she really wants to have an important discussion with him, take a drive. As both of you ride along with your eyes focused on the road ahead, the child with Asperger's may be much more comfortable than if you were sitting across the table from him establishing eye contact during the conversation. Sure enough, as they drove home, she noticed that, indeed, Jason was much more talkative than in a face-to-face setting. From that point on, whenever she had something important to discuss with him, they went for a drive.

Dr. B: Although children with autism could be blind or deaf, those anomalies are not specifically associated as characteristics of autism. However, as sight and hearing are two of our senses, and children with autism often have sensory issues, we must consider the effects of sights and sounds in our environment. Children with autism are often fascinated with visual stimuli. They may enjoy staring at a toy or other object for long periods of time, looking at it from different angles. They may enjoy watching the water running into the sink. I have seen children who love to stare at their shadows on the playground. They may show an intense fascination with things that spin or move in certain patterns. Having a compulsion to spin the wheels on a toy car is an example of this. Rather than play with the car in the same manner as a typical child, he may take more enjoyment in watching the wheels spin for long periods of time. Another odd trait of children with autism is that they often seem to look at things with their peripheral vision rather than looking at them straight on. Some parents of children on the spectrum say their child "looks right through people" as opposed to looking *at* them. Changes in the child's visual perception of his environment may cause an unwanted reaction. If things don't look the way he expects them to, he may get very upset.

If the parents or teachers intend to use any visual supports to help the child, they first need to know how the child reacts to visual stimuli. The way the child processes something he sees may be different from our visual perception of the same object. Five-year-old Grant drew a picture of a lady and proudly showed it to his mother, who asked, "Oh, is this Mommy?"

"No, Mommy, it's Ms. Lauren. Ms. Lauren is the only one who has stars in her eyes. Can't you see them, Mommy?" Sure enough, a closer look at the picture showed that he had drawn the stars he alone sees when he looks at Miss Lauren's eyes.

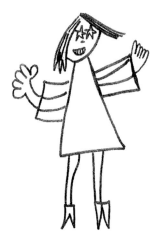

Miss Lauren with stars in her eyes

Some children are strongly affected by colors. Many typically developing children have a favorite color, but children with autism often take this to the extreme, becoming obsessed with a certain color. In my experience, blue, orange, or black seem to be the colors of obsession most often.

Mrs. Luck: I have had two children fanatically obsessed with the color blue. Teachers would use this knowledge to motivate them. When they refused to do their work using a different color pencil or crayon, a blue marker would inspire them. Blue incentives were used. I had a student teacher who wore blue shirts, arranged blue chairs, and brought in blue incentives as rewards when working with Tyler, who desperately loved blue. She had him wrapped around her little finger, so to speak. He loved her and would work hard to please her. Tyler's parents told me that they used his love of the color blue at home in their behavior management plan. If Tyler started having a meltdown, they quietly started removing the blue knick-knacks from the room. He knew he could earn the blue objects back by showing good behavior.

Mrs. Nic: I have actually had two students obsessed with orange. You could depend on the fact that they would each have on an orange shirt every day and carry an orange backpack and lunchbox. Orange objects seemed to keep them in a happy mood. If the orange object were misplaced or forgotten at home, the mood would change. The parents and I felt this was a fairly simple thing we could do for these children, and it really didn't hurt anything to attempt to flood their environment with colors that made them feel good.

Shelli: Joshuah is affected by the color-specific issue. He is very aware of the color of things, especially when it comes to food labels. He has an idea in his head of what the packaging of certain item should look like, and if we switch to a different brand, he won't eat it.

Dr. B: Typical children can be somewhat fussy eaters, and even most adults have some foods we just prefer not to eat. A parent may find that a child with autism might have many contributing factors can lead to extreme food selectivity. It may be so extreme that nutrition and health issues arise. Some children just refuse to eat or eat only tiny amounts for days, then return to their normal routine. This extreme food selectivity is well beyond what we would call fussy eating. When this happens, we first want to rule out an underlying illness or dental problems. Various medications may also have an effect on hunger and may have an effect on the eating patterns of children.

The child might have an enhanced sense of smell, which may change his food enjoyment.

Mrs. Luck: Twelve-year-old Tim likes to sniff the back shoulder of people who interact with him. He is especially delighted if they have on a sleeveless shirt. He seems happier when he can sniff the shoulder of females than males. After sniffing, he taps the back of his hand to his nose twice, then walks away.

Mrs. Nic: My family was traveling by air last summer, and there was a family in the boarding area with a preteen son who displayed autistic characteristics. Obviously stressed by the travel experience, he was intent on sniffing the hair of the people around him, especially the children. His sister complained loudly to the parents, "Mom! Ben is smelling my hair again!"

Dr. B: Sensory issues are certainly at the core of some of the extreme food preferences we see in children on the spectrum. They may be extremely sensitive to certain tastes or possibly oblivious to other tastes that a typical person would find rather offensive. Foods with certain textures may give them pleasure, while other textures almost seem painful to them. The same is true of food temperatures.

Mrs. Luck: Eleven-year-old Tony brings a whole onion in his lunch every day. Not a sweet Vidalia onion but a strong, pungent onion. The odor fills the school as lunches are served. He just chews it down and loves it. By the way, he *hates* peaches!

Elizabeth: If your child is hyposensitive to tastes, it is vital that you keep harmful substances put away. In a sense, you may have experienced a touch of this when you have had a cold and food loses its taste.

Dr. B: Humans have a variety of specific taste buds that allow them to perceive different tastes. There are four basic types of taste buds: those designed to detect salty, sour, bitter, or sweet. A child with autism may be hypersensitive to tastes and choose to only eat foods from one of these categories. To assure a nutritious, varied diet, parents get very creative with condiments. Selectivity and routine can also cross over into eating issues. We have seen children who will only eat foods that are a certain color or served from a favorite plate. Parents find themselves becoming food detectives to discover the root of the eating problem.

Shelli: We struggle with food so much. My oldest will not eat very many foods at all. He likes one thing really well for a while and then gets burned out on it, and he looks for something else that he likes really well. I used to make him six scrambled eggs for breakfast. He would bring me the pan I made them in, and he would get out the eggs and cheese. He was so cute. For a while, I was the only one who could make them for him. This speaks to his need for sameness. He is the most rigid about having things always remain the same. The temperature of the food has to be just right, or he would hand it back to me, or he would put it in the microwave himself. Needless to say, he is a big help in the kitchen because he likes to make sure I am making things correctly. If he sees that I have not fixed him something he wants for dinner, he takes my hand to the door because he is ready to leave. He thinks we need to go to the store or pick him up some food in a drive-thru (which I hate doing). I have come to this understanding by trial and error. He would have the worst meltdowns over these types of things. My youngest is almost the exact opposite. She eats anything if she is hungry.

Mrs. Nic: Michelle, a teenager, would only eat food that matched the color of clothing she wore that day. If she knew the family was going out for pizza, she would change into a reddish-orange sweater. If she went to a restaurant wearing a white sweater, she would only order clam chowder, fettuccini, or mashed potatoes with cream gravy. If she did not have availability to food to match the outfit, she would rather not eat at all.

Mrs. Luck: We have quite a few students with autism who cannot eat foods that are touching another food on the plate. They would eat any of the items served separately, but if it touches another food item, they can't stand that.

Elizabeth: If your child is eating only hard-boiled eggs (and of course, refuses to finish it if the yolk falls out), this needs to be called to the attention of your occupational therapist. Behaviors of this type may also be because of tactile (touch) sensitivities in the mouth, which your speech-language pathologist can help you address.

Dr. B: The sense of touch is another area where this population differs from typical children. I have seen several children who obviously liked feeling a smooth wall or a smooth wooden railing. Not so pleasurable is the texture of shaving cream or mud. Many don't like the feeling of going barefoot. While typical children may love to finger-paint, the idea might be conflicting for the children with autism who would like to paint but do not want to touch the paint. Those with higher language skills may ask you if you could please bring them a paintbrush to use in the finger-painting project. Some children will have an aversion to some articles of clothing based on the textures and will avoid wearing certain materials due to that sensation. This even extends to likes and dislikes for certain foods based entirely on the textures.

Elizabeth: Even the perception of pain may be different for our children. It is common for children with ASD to lack appropriate response to pain or even to be insensitive to pain. Nicole was one of these children. She seemed to be immune to pain. I recall one experience when Nicole fell and began to cry. I swiftly went to her side and comforted her. I remember a woman spoke up and said, "Well, if you cater to her like that you will teach her to be needy and want attention." In disbelief of what I heard I replied, "My child doesn't cry unless she is really hurting and it is a joy for me to be able to comfort her." This woman didn't know it was incredibly rare that my child cried in pain, and even less common that she let me comfort her. I was going to enjoy every second.

Dr. B: Sometimes, he may seem to not even feel pain at all, and another time, he might seem hypersensitive to the same stimulus. Some physicians have attributed this to a basic inconsistency in the neural responses.

Along with the commonly identified senses of hearing, sight, smell, touch, and vision, children with autism may also have difficulties with the vestibular and proprioceptive senses. Vestibular refers to the sense of our bodies in relation to the earth's surface. They may have little sense of themselves in relation to the space around them. Proprioceptive refers to the awareness of their own limbs to their body.

Elizabeth: When we receive sensory input from the world around us, our brains usually unconsciously translate this input into meaning and produce a reaction. So what our bodies experience affects what we do. A child with autism will not react as we would typically expect. Luckily, there are things you can do to help your child overcome hypersensitivities and hyposensitivities to the various stimuli.

For instance, if an individual is hypersensitive to a certain stimulus when exposed at a minimal level, slowly increasing the intensity will help to desensitize him. The idea is not unlike building taste tolerance for a disliked but necessary nutritional supplement—or even broccoli. A child with autism may not like to have sticky hands and might have meltdowns when he gets the smallest amount of food on his fingers. Expose him to minimal discomfort and increase that exposure over time. Do activities that require touching objects or substances. What once seemed too much is now okay. And tomorrow that new level of comfort will be challenged.

If an individual is experiencing hyposensitivities, the stimulus he is receiving is not enough to create satisfaction or a typical response. This often looks like behavior issues. Why does a child with autism not respond or seek out excessive stimulation? Because they lack what most of us feel from the environment. To help an individual with hyposensitivities, adequate stimulation must be present in his life. Teach your child to seek out appropriate ways and times for that stimulation. If your child is hyposensitive to touch, deep pressure activities like rolling a therapy ball over his body may increase his knowledge of being touched. Increasing exposure may help an individual become more sensitive to a given stimulus.

Interestingly enough, both types of sensitivities will most likely be present in each individual with autism. When working with someone with sensitivities issues, look at his individual traits. Is he pushing his limits to reach new things in his life? Is increased exposure helping the child cope, or is it encouraging autistic behaviors? Pay careful attention to your child's behavior; it will be your guide.

Social Skills

Dr. B: During childhood, youngsters learn to interact socially with others. This is one of the most important tasks of the early years. Forging friendships with other children as well as with adults is based on successful social interactions. Lessons learned at an early age teach us how to live with others in our environment throughout our lives. These friendships serve many purposes for us as we grow up. Our peers become our support group, our source of humor, pleasure, and social learning. Our friends help us cope with stress, anxiety, and new situations. Children with special needs of any sort often seem to need extra guidance in developing and maintaining friendships and in dealing with others socially.

By definition, children on the autism spectrum have difficulty with social interactions. They may display deficits in nonverbal behaviors such as eye-to-eye gaze, facial expression, and gestures we normally use to regulate social interaction. They may fail to develop peer relationships at their appropriate developmental level. We often see a lack of spontaneously seeking to share enjoyment and poor social or emotional reciprocity. In our classrooms for children who struggle with social adjustment, we formally teach social skills that typical children pick up on their own. Children with autism need to be taught the social skills that come much more naturally to their peers. We teach them to read facial features and body language. They must be shown how to initiate a social interaction and how to respond when another person begins a contact with them. They can learn how to respond to the emotions of others, but this does not come naturally to them. Showing an interest in other children must be nurtured and friendship skills need to be fostered.

Elizabeth: One of the best therapies Nicole did was Jessica. Jessica was a friend. She was a neighbor girl who was an only child. Needing someone to play with while her mother studied after attending graduate school all day, Jessica found her way to our home. She was a couple of years older, which made her quite predictable. Nicole and Jessica played side by side for many months. Then parallel play gave way to interacting, then turn taking. Bonding came slowly, but Nicole's needs brought out the nurturing side of this young girl, and out of compassion, friendship was formed.

Dr. B: Difficulty in social interaction is a problem that needs to be addressed from both sides. In order for the child to be able communicate more successfully, we as educators and parents work to help not only the child on the spectrum but also those who interact with him. My granddaughter, Courtney, came home from school last week and told us about what seemed to be sensitivity training on the topic of autism in her sixth-grade classroom. She said that as the teacher was explaining autism to the class, one boy, Frankie, jumped up and happily announced to the class, "I have Asperger's syndrome." She said Frankie went on to tell the class about what that means, mentioning the things that are hard for him, but especially detailing the many special talents he has. She seemed pretty impressed about Frankie's special talents.

Many children can benefit from structured "social skills classes." In formal settings, children learn social expectations that typical children learn without formal instruction. Social skills classes normally cover topics such as how to form and maintain friendships, the dynamics of a conversation, and development of play skills. Instruction in social skills classes may be a combination of direct instruction and role playing to practice the skill they are working on that day. These classes cover such topics as how to cope with conflict and how to deal with your own emotions. It would be appropriate for them to learn about empathy for others and how to recognize and deal with the emotions of others. On the TV sitcom *Big Bang Theory*, Sheldon has obviously memorized social rules of etiquette and does his best to enforce those rules in various situations. When one of the other characters is upset, Sheldon often recites and enforces the rule, "Social etiquette dictates that when a friend is upset, you should offer them a hot beverage" all the while making it clear he really does not sympathize with the plight of the friend.

Mrs. Luck: Problems with social skills include a lack of perspective of others, poor command of conversational expectations, poor eye contact, lack of understanding humor, and modeling behaviors after adults rather than children. A boy who I had in class a couple of years ago came into my room during evening open house this week. He walked into my room, sat down, and said "Hello, Mrs. Luck." He then talked nonstop for about five minutes, telling me all about a Disney movie he had been watching a lot lately. Then he stood up and announced, "I'm finished. Good-bye, Mrs. Luck" and walked out of my room.

Shelli: Socially, my daughter is so passive about a lot of things. Some would say this is a good thing but not always. While my son pushes his environment to understand him, she is content to just sit back in her own world. She will play by herself for hours, and I never have to worry about her. When it comes time for us to get her to do things for us, she pushes away. We struggled with her therapies in the beginning because she was content just to sit on my lap the whole time. If she didn't want to do the shape-sorter or some other task being asked of her, she would have an awful meltdown. Nothing we did would make her calm down. She was done.

Mrs. Nic: This population seems socially naive compared to age-matched peers in the classroom. For example, they are more likely to innocently reach up and touch the teacher's breasts as they are talking to her. They actually need to be taught not to touch others inappropriately, whereas the typical child already has that concept pretty firmly in their mind by the time they come to school.

Possibly because they are so literal in their thinking, they often do not understand jokes or *kidding*. When someone kids them, they often take the statement for reality.

Dr. B: The older students in our school had been discussing the book *How to Eat Fried Worms*. The students really enjoyed their introduction to the age-appropriate book. In an attempt to bring interest and humor to the class, the teachers staged a little joke. They rolled Tootsie Rolls into worm shapes and showed them to the class and ate them, all the while giggling and winking. A fifteen-year-old boy with autism started to cry. As the teachers kiddingly urged the class to try one, this boy had a total meltdown. The teachers immediately told the class they were eating Tootsie Rolls, not really worms, and that the children could play this joke on their parents when they got home that night. Even the explanation did not calm the upset boy. The rest of the class howled with laughter at the little prank. They talked the rest of the day about the great joke the teachers played on them.

The lack of a sense of humor may extend to adulthood. I was giving a tour of the Center for Autism to a high-functioning college student, Jacob, and his mother. We happened upon Braden, a little three-year-old who is super cute and very bright. We enjoyed interacting with Braden for a few minutes, after which I remarked to Jacob's mom, "I would just like to put Braden in my pocket and take that little guy home with me." The mom smiled and nodded in agreement. Jacob, taking my statement literally, quickly informed me, "Oh no, that will never work. I see you have a preference for denim jeans. Since the standard width of a pocket on denim jeans is 8.9 centimeters, that child will never fit in your pocket."

Mrs. Luck: Another characteristic we see as both a positive and a negative is that children with autism do not lie. It just is not something they would ever consider. While as parents and teachers we see this as a wonderful attribute for a child to have, it can also cause discomfort. These are the kids who say to the teacher, "Wow, you are really old" or innocently tell a classmate, "You are fat." They may look at the picture a classmate has just painted and honestly assure her it is really ugly. They aren't saying those things to be mean. They are just being honest beyond the point that is socially acceptable. An important thing for parents and teachers to remember is while they always tell the truth, it is *the truth as they see it*. Their perception of the truth about something may be a step away from reality, but they tell it as they see it. That *truth* might not always match our perception of a fact. As George Costanza on the sitcom *Seinfeld* says, "It's not a lie if you believe it."

Dr. B: Opportunities for children to develop the skills needed for social success are more limited for the child with autism. A typically developing child may be taken to the park where he easily joins a group of other children at play. They make friends easily and quickly get to know one another. A mother named Kimberly told me why she does not expose her son Jeremy, age five, to those social situations. She is tired of the judgmental looks she gets from other parents that do not understand her family's struggles. She has quickly come to the point of not wanting to form friendships with other families except those having children with autism. She said she will have other adult friends. She will go to dinner with these adults, and she will socialize elsewhere with them. However, she will not discuss her children with the parents of the neuro-typical children. She will no longer invite them or their families to her home because they "just don't understand." The only children she will invite for a play date, or accept a play date with, are those from other families that have children on the spectrum. She feels that the only people who are not judgmental of her and her children are the other families who have children with autism. Upon hearing Kimberly's description of the need for these families to network with each other, we took that into consideration and built in some family social time each day during school dismissal. The children are allowed to play in the sensory area while the parents are free to compare notes and chat with other parents who understand what they are going through. Parents of children with common characteristics can benefit from hearing the experiences of the other families. They share coping strategies or just offer a word of support. They delight together in the small steps of success of the other children in the group.

Lower-functioning or nonverbal children with autism may spend much of their time engaged in solitary play and may even adjust their body posture to exclude others from their personal space. When given a toy, they often prefer to stare at the toy, especially if it has a moving part. If they are given a toy car, a typically developing child usually runs it on an imaginary road on the table or floor. However, when a child with autism is presented with a toy car, he may prefer to look at it from different angles and perhaps spin the tires. This object does not seem to necessarily represent a car but is rather a delightful object of its own accord. Play and the formation of relationships are important to child development. It has been said, "Play is the work of children,"[11] and children who do not have play skills are at a disadvantage in development of language and cognitive skills.

Shelli: We like to take our kids to the park. Joshuah sometimes will want another child to play with him, maybe go down the slide, and because he does not use words, he will gently put his hands on the other child's shoulders and try to move him to where he wants him to go. I must also mention that these are usually younger kids. It really makes those kids' parents so nervous. They are afraid Joshuah is going to hurt their child. For me, it is the cutest thing. It is really hard for Joshuah to even touch them because he really doesn't like doing it. Touching them is all he has at times. It is awkward for him, but like I said, it is super cute to see.

Mrs. Luck: The fact that Asperger's kids are very literal and often don't understand abstract language deeply affects their social skills. An example of this struggle is the concept of "friends." I had a third-grade student who had been diagnosed with Asperger's syndrome. He was on the higher-functioning end of the autism spectrum. He told his mother, "I don't have any friends." At first, I thought this was a social skills problem and arranged for other students to play with him at recess. Still, we heard, "I have no friends." Then I asked him, "What is a friend?" and he said he did not know, but everyone else seemed to have one and he didn't. I explained friends were the kids you walked to speech with, talked to in the classroom, and played with at recess. He looked at me and said "Okay, I have lots of friends."

Mrs. Nic: Another interesting feature of their play is that it can be amazingly repetitive. When Newton plays, he always goes to the area with all the blocks. He builds the exact same tower, using the same blocks, over and over. He seems perfectly content with that limited, solitary play behavior.

Dr. B: Preferring to be alone is one of the most common traits of those with ASD. Since they show little connection to those around them, this may be perceived as the person being aloof. Sometimes, they just don't care to interact. Other times, it may be that they would like to interact but don't know how. Some have postulated that the sensory input is so delayed in these children that they don't actually *hear* what another person says until it is too late to reply meaningfully. This is confirmed by the fact that the child may not even startle when there is a loud noise that would normally produce that reaction.

The extreme end of social adjustment is aggression. When children show aggression, it may be toward other children, toward adults, toward themselves, or toward objects, such as toys. It must be dealt with in a consistent manner and at an early point before it escalates to a dangerous level. If the object of the aggression tends to be other children, every precaution must be taken to keep the other children safe from the aggressor. Some aggressive behaviors are the manifestation of not having a verbal capability to express anger and frustration. Other behaviors may be attention seeking. We need to be careful not to feed those behaviors by actually giving the child the attention he is seeking. In extreme cases, a good behavior analyst can provide a helpful behavior plan. The crux of any good behavior plan is that it must be followed by all persons of authority in the child's environment.

Mrs. Luck: Behavior problems I have seen stem from either a lack of understanding that their behaviors impact others, difficulty differentiating fact from fiction, or being very gullible.

Shelli: Violent behaviors are really scary to every parent. At times, you feel so helpless. There was a time we struggled so much with Joshuah's sleeping. He hadn't slept in over three days. Nights were awful, and I dreaded bedtime. Joshuah would get so hyper at bedtime. It was like his body would amp up, and the less sleep he got, the more violent he got. He would bang his little head into to the walls with such force, laugh about it, then run full speed across the room, and bash his head all over again. My baby was so tired. I knew he was, but I couldn't hold him or rock him to sleep. He wouldn't let me touch him. I had been calling our doctor for the past couple of days, and they had nothing to tell me. By day three, I was so exhausted, I decided I would lock Joshuah in his room, so I could sleep. I didn't feel like I could actually sleep with him screaming and banging his head against the wall, but I needed a break. Moments after he was in his room, I heard a loud crash and then my son crying. I ran into the room and found the bookshelf pushed over on top of him. I removed the bookshelf and the books to pick him up. I checked his head, his eyes, and before I knew it, he was asleep. I feared he had a concussion. I called our doctor, and they instructed me to call 911. Before long, I was with paramedics trying to wake my son. It took me pinching his leg, and he woke up crying. They looked him over and assured me there was no concussion, no broken bones—he was fine. They told me the extreme adrenaline rush must have made him sleepy enough to finally go to sleep. I called my doctor then, very upset, and pleaded that I need him to sleep. I needed to know what I could give him. We were then told to try Melatonin. It works great for us. Joshuah needs it every night. Clonidine also helps him. He now sleeps through the night, and he hasn't tried hurting himself since.

Dr. B: Another upsetting characteristic is fear. It is normal for young children to have fears, such as being afraid of the dark. A certain amount of fear is healthy and serves a purpose. Children with autism have the added burden of irrational fears. They are often terrorized by an object or event that is normally not seen as something to fear. In contrast, many times they have no fear of things they should be afraid of. I have heard of children terrified of flies, people sneezing, and Scooby-Doo on the cartoon. A child who may have no fear of running out into a busy street may be deathly afraid of a baby duck in a petting zoo.

Elizabeth: What may seem like irrational fears may not be so strange if we understand what is causing those fears or, more precisely, what is being interpreted as scary. Nathan had a phase where he seemed terrified to walk through doors, showing fear as we dragged him across thresholds. In talking with his older sister, she had a different interpretation of the situation. She remembers behaving in similar fashion. She didn't want to walk through doors after people she didn't like. She didn't want to get their "stuff" on her. She walked through a separate door, waited for someone else to pass through the door to cleanse it, or leaned far to the side to miss the offending person's aura. So we began to understand that Nathan did not want to avoid going to school, but that maybe there was something else, especially since we saw this behavior in all situations, not just school. We did seem to find that it was more of a predictability issue with Nathan. As we began to help him understand what would happen if he passed through the door, we saw his anxiety diminish and his success increase.

For obvious fears, we help to provide coping techniques and strategies. Both Nicole and Chase feared flies. Their flight patterns embodied unpredictability. With Nicole, we helped her learn to use the words, "Shoo, fly, don't bother me." Giving her words helped her release the anxiety and face the vicious beasts. With Chase, more invasive action had to be employed. We bought some fake flies and a fly swatter and practiced controlling the situation. While I don't know if he ever killed a real fly, he learned that he was bigger and stronger than the opposing foe, giving him the confidence to face his fears.

Dr. B: One common stimulus that elicits terror among this population is a loud or sudden noise. Parents may carry noise-reducing headphones similar to the type used industrially if they know they will be exposed to loud noises.

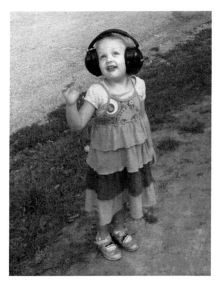

Izzy enjoying the outdoors wearing noise-reducing earphones

Strange or new places are often described as fear-producing for kids with autism. Many are afraid of the dark. Some have night terrors, making it difficult for them or their families to sleep. Higher-functioning people on the spectrum have labeled *fear* as the primary emotion of people with ASD. Fortunately, parents I have talked to feel that the terrors do lessen somewhat as the child ages. At the very least, they tell me the terrors do not worsen as the child gets older. Often, the ASD child's fears are so great they resemble phobias.

Some young people are quite open about the fear of germs and disease. Recently, I spent some time with John, a bright high school student who refers to himself as an Aspie. His mother accompanied him when we met, and she served as his social coach. When we were being introduced, she quietly prompted him to look me in the eye. He immediately complied, even though it was fleeting and was obviously uncomfortable for him. She then prompted him to shake my hand. He took a quick breath, held it in, and extended his hand. It reminded me of a youngster about to jump off the high dive, taking a breath to shore up his bravery. I accepted his outreached hand and shook it politely. I could see him mentally counting the seconds, and when he reached five, he dropped my hand, and quickly began rubbing his hand on his shirt, in what appeared to be his attempt to erase any possible germs until he could sanitize his hands. As they left my office, she allowed him to use a liquid hand sanitizer, which I am sure made him feel much better. Part of the job of the families and the educators of children on the spectrum is to help them cope with their fears, and that can take many forms, depending on the individual.

Mrs. Luck: My best advice to parents and teachers is to not transmit your own fears to the child. Children are highly sensitive and will pick up on both your verbal and your nonverbal indicators. When we would take children to the pool, a few moms would remark about their own terror of the water. They would tell how they are so happy the children will learn to swim, while stressing that they themselves have always been frightened of the water. They would be obviously nervous about putting the child down to walk to the pool with the other children. Inevitably, after hearing of their mothers' fears, those same children would be terrorized by the experience. Seeing Mom's distressed face peering in the viewing window validated the child's fear. The child, learning water is something

Mom fears, assumes it is something evil that he should be afraid of also.

Shelli: Joshuah has always sought out heights. No fear. At the age of two, he climbed to the top of our shop building, and I could not get him down. I had to call my husband. On the other hand, he is afraid of walking into a room that has a handful of people in it, even when he knows all the people in the room.

Dr. B: A child's social adjustment might be judged by other people based on the physical contact he demonstrates. Children with ASD seem to either totally avoid physical contact, or they crave it. I have seen children who are uncomfortable with physical contact who enroll in a very nurturing program where they are heavily reinforced for physical contact, and they soon take delight in the hugging and touching. A small private school I was associated with where children were conditioned to truly enjoy human contact was purchased by a large corporation from the east coast. The large corporation had been exposed to a high incidence of litigation in the eastern states and was nervous about the children in this school receiving hugs and tickles from the staff. So the corporation that bought the school placed restrictions on that manner of touching. The children continued to ask for the hugs and tickles from the staff, and the parents felt that a very valuable reinforcement tool had been taken away. They felt that the warmth that came from the teachers was one reason for the strong success of the school. This was in contrast to the previous experiences of the national firm, which found litigation to be plentiful and costly. Both the parents and the national directors wanted the best for the children, but coming from vastly different backgrounds, they had different ideas of how to provide the best care.

For a baby to shun parental physical contact is heartbreaking. Some infants are just apathetic to the touch of the parent. Others babies stiffen up when the parent picks him up. We normally think of the parent's touch as something that would comfort an upset baby, but here we sometimes have the opposite scenario—a contented baby who resists and cries when the parent attempts to hold him. With the cuddling time being thought of as so important for the building of the relationship between parent and baby, a baby's rejection of human touch may cause negative feelings in the parent.

Elizabeth: It's hard to know sometimes if a child actually does not like touch or if he really does not even feel it. Sometimes, you will see a child who resists cuddling if initiated by another but enjoys cuddling on his own terms.

Dr. B: So for a variety of reasons, some children with autism seriously enjoy cuddling, and others would rather not. I have seen children make a total turn-around on this after attending school where touch is paired with things the student enjoys. If the child loves Thomas the Tank Engine, the teacher might progressively touch him on the arm when the Thomas video is played. If he loves juice, she may serve him snack while touching him on the back. Over time, the children learn to enjoy touch as it is associated with pleasant things. Parents and teachers I know agree that children on the spectrum prefer a firm solid touch as opposed to a light, feathery touch. Children have explained that the light touch feels like it is a shock, while the firm pressure feels comforting and calming.

In 2010, HBO made a movie about the life of Temple Grandin, now a well-known animal scientist, lecturer, and author living with autism. She actually built a "hugging machine" to give herself mechanical hugs when she needed that pressure and sensation. I have visited some autism programs that have purchased commercial devices similar to that invention. When children are feeling stressed, they can go to the squeezing machines and calm themselves.

Often children with autism perseverate on certain behaviors, thoughts, or topics of conversation. *Perseverating* means they produce certain words or actions over and over, such as repeating a phrase, flapping arms, shutting a door, turning a light on and off, flicking fingers, lining up objects, rubbing hands together, or spinning objects. Parents have described these actions as perhaps replacing the play of a typically developing child because the child with autism may have no play skills to pass his time. To an observer, the behaviors seem to be odd and meaningless, self-stimulating, and ritualistic. This would describe thirteen-year-old Allen who has eaten two corn dogs every day for lunch for the last three years. It would also describe seven-year-old Frankie who has insisted on coming to school every day dressed as Sponge Bob, or Aiden, who wears a plastic police vest every day.

Action-related perseveration is common in the form of rocking or pacing. Eleven-year-old Jaime runs two steps, flicks her fingers, bends over in laughter, then walks the rest of the way every time she ambulates across the room. Another example of action-related perseveration is displayed by Jonah, a high school student. He asks people for a high five all day. For Jaime and Jonah, it seems that the perseverated action serves to attain desired sensory stimuli.

Topic-related perseverations can remain with a child for years. Jonah perseverates on the topic of Chuck-E Cheese. This didn't seem inappropriate when he was six, but now that he is fourteen, it accentuates the differences between him and his age-matched peers, and that behavior has become an embarrassment to his family. As with many children on the spectrum, Jonah's perseverations become more intense with stress, or as he gets more stimulated.

Besides calling unwanted attention to the child, perseverations can interfere with other thoughts and even block learning from taking place. There does seem to be a trend in children with Asperger's to reduce the perseverations or to modify them to be more socially acceptable as the child grows into adolescence. They learn to shelter or hide the action from the judgment of the viewer.

Perseveration can sometimes be an attribute. We saw a television news story of a boy with autism who worked on the sidelines with his high school basketball team. On his own, he tirelessly practiced shooting baskets. When the coach finally put him into the game, his hours of basketball practice paid off, and he became a star for the night. More recently, a TV news story spotlighted Anthony Starego, a high school boy with autism who is a kicker on his school football team. His dad tells that as a young boy, Anthony obsessively watched a video of a college kicker kicking a field goal. Now he delighted the nation with the news clip showing him successfully kicking a field goal to win the game. In the postgame interview, Anthony explained that he practices kicking the field goal over and over. His coach said he has practiced the kick thousands of times. If practice makes perfect, children on the spectrum can indeed become perfect at an activity because their attention to it may not waver. His dad explains that Anthony's heightened ability to break an activity into its requisite parts, along with his dedication to repeating the activity, proved a winning combination for him. [12]

Many people hate change and stick to routines in their own way. Those on the spectrum just seem to have taken this intolerance for change to the extreme. Their need for routine is intense and extreme.

Another way in which children on the spectrum differ socially involves imagination. Imagination is in our heads, so how do we know if someone has imagination? It is often claimed that children with autism do not have imaginations. All we can safely assume is that the child with autism usually does not exhibit the same signs of imaginative play as other children. Typically developing children will watch how other children play with toys and will imitate the other children. They will pick up both the good and the bad traits they observe in others. For example, if you give a typically developing child a set of blocks, the child might choose to line up blocks one next to the other the first time you present the blocks to him. When the typically developing child sees others build with the blocks, he will start to build with them also, imitating the play behavior he sees. A child with autism may not even notice others are playing with the blocks at all, and he may not spontaneously imitate that behavior.

Typical children may express their imagination through their art from an early age. Justin's mom explained the sadness she and her husband felt at not sharing in her child's little art creations like other parents do. The walls of their refrigerator held no pictures created by his little hands. One day, Justin was on the potty, and she went to check on him. He had smeared his feces on the wall. When she looked at the wall, instead of being horrified, she was transfixed by the patterns and design she saw. She and her husband took pictures of Justin's artwork that was smeared on the wall. They printed the pictures and proudly hung them on the refrigerator. Visitors to the home see the "finger-painting" done by their son and are unaware of the unorthodox materials he used to create the picture.

Mrs. Luck: When we bought a new game of Angry Birds for the integrated kindergarten class, both Gordon and Josiah were perfectly happy to sit and line up the little plastic birds. Then a third child, Derek, joined the game and knew how to catapult the little birds in the slingshot. The slingshot trick immediately became Gordon's activity of choice when playing with this toy. Josiah, who has autism, continued to merely line up the birds, never imitating the slingshot game.

Mrs. Nic: In my kindergarten class, when the children all get involved in symbolic play, such as playing house or store or school, the children on the spectrum do not join in. At that point, they gravitate away from the group and usually entertain themselves examining a small object. With some help and guidance, they seem to be able to learn to play with the toy food, but they don't seem to just pick it up from watching other kids.

Dr. B: On the other end of this continuum are kids who have so much imagination that they live in a fantasy world. The children who get locked into that pretend world seem often to be the kids with Asperger's syndrome. Robert is a sixteen-year-old who firmly believes all the L.A. Lakers are his brothers. He brags to everyone and relates fully constructed scenarios about his home life with his "brothers." Even though he cannot drive, he has an active imagination about his adventures as a race car driver. According to him, he even builds his own race cars. If we question him about facts in the story, he digs in deeper. Another boy in that class, Tim, believes he lives on *Leave it to Beaver* and even insists on calling his teacher Ms. Landers. Yet another student, Jason, is convinced he is one of the *Brady Bunch*. If you ask him the names of his brothers and sisters, he tells you without hesitation, "Cindy, Jan, Greg, Marcia, Peter, and Bobby." He tells delightful antics each day of his housekeeper, Alice.

Mrs. Luck: In contrast to that, Xander is an example of a typically developing boy with a more normal imagination. An example of how he could be talked down happened just this morning. He told me he had eaten three cases of toothpaste last night. I questioned him.

"Three cases…really…three cases. So that would be about seventy-five tubes of toothpaste?"

"Well, maybe it was three tubes."

"Three whole tubes or just part of each tube?"

"Well, maybe one tube."

"Okay, are you sure? A whole tube?"

"Yes, I'm sure. Mom said I could."

"Okay, just wanted to get the facts ready for my report."

"What report?"

"The one I give to the EMTs when they get here with the ambulance."

"Well, maybe it was just the toothpaste I put on my toothbrush. Do you still need to write a report?"

"Nope, all kids do that."

The difference between Xander and the other three boys is that Xander really knew he was telling a whopper and could be talked down.

Elizabeth: Fantasy is something I have struggled with when helping my children develop functional skills. I love the creative aspect, but I know firsthand that individuals with autism often use it to escape, to rest from this world. Using it for productive endeavors can be an asset, but giving into a fantasy world and living there is something we as parents must learn to recognize.

Dr. B: While some unusual behaviors may be harmless, others may present a danger to the child or to others. Children and adults with autism may engage in self-injurious behaviors (also known as SIB). Self-injurious behaviors are simply any actions the child performs that result in physical injury to his own body. Types of self-injury behaviors might include hitting, biting, excessively scratching, or picking at himself. These are not accidental injuries but rather are purposeful attacks on his own body. The magnitude may range from an outburst of rage to a barely noticeable yet incessant behavior. People with these tendencies seem to show a preference for one particular SIB inflicted upon one particular body part. When parents and teachers talk about the behavior, they often describe a behavior that the child does not "outgrow." Unfortunately, it seems to continue and become more severe unless it is treated. In my experience, SIBs are difficult to simply redirect.

Self-injurious behaviors seem to have more than one possible motivation. Some children may resort to hurting themselves rather than striking out at others when they are in a rage. When Joel gets angry at a peer or a teacher, he hits himself. Others seem to head bang or hurt themselves in a search for self-stimulation. Still another group of children injure themselves in an effort to calm themselves when they are excited. A fourth group exhibits these behaviors as an attention-seeking activity. When Keisha does not have the immediate attention of her preferred teacher, she bangs her head hard against the wall and starts to cry. This is certainly her way of taking the attention from the child who is working with the favorite teacher and bringing the adult's attention to herself. Now, when it is not Keisha's turn with the preferred staff member, she wears a helmet and works at a desk in front of a mat on the wall.

Parents are certainly justified in their concern over this destructive behavior. Among the most dangerous types of SIB is head banging. A child may violently bang his head against any fixed object, such as a wall or a table. I knew a nine-year-old named Jesse who engaged in violent head banging. He preferred abusing his forehead. His tool of choice was any coat hook on the wall. When he would enter a new location, you could see him visually scan the area for wall hooks. At his first opportunity, he would dash for the hooks and bash his forehead into them. When he enrolled at our program, we prepared the path from the bus to his classroom by removing everything from the hallway. We then prepared his classroom by installing mats on the wall in his area. The coat hooks were moved to a level too high for him to reach. We couldn't remove the desire, but we could make our environment as safe for him as it could be.

Mrs. Luck: Doug is sixteen years old and gets very excited during play. He has large pink calluses on his hands from biting his own hands when he gets excited. It seems to allow him to calm himself when he is overstimulated.

Mrs. Nic: Five-year-old Lexi would gouge her mosquito bites until they bled and became horribly large open sores. Her parents would cover them with Band-Aids and send a box of extra Band-Aids to school to cover the wounds when she pulled the original Band-Aids off. She was very adept at sneaking the Band-Aid off and digging at the sores. We would have to continually be cleaning blood off her hands and around the bites. As we would be washing the blood from under her fingernails on her right hand, her left hand would dart into the sore and violently dig. To help in the effort, her parents started sending her in long-sleeved shirts and long pants, even on hot days, to try to keep her from opening the sores. Taking our eyes off of Lexi for one minute would result in her getting her hands beneath the clothing and scratching off the scabs. Her obsession with those sores lasted throughout the summer and was a true battle for the parents and the teacher.

Dr. B: David, an exasperated father, sat in my office last spring. His son who is going to high school was creating large bald spots by pulling out tufts of his own hair—all from the left side of his head. David's frustration was obvious as we searched for the solution. "I try distracting him, begging him, even taking away privileges, but he keeps pulling the hair out. I am thrilled he is actually learning to read and do math, but what good does that do if we can't get a grip on these bizarre behaviors?" Then as we brainstormed, we zeroed in on the fact that this boy was a strong rule follower. He had told me in the past, "Rules are my best friend." I brought him into my office and told him we now have a rule against students pulling out their own hair. He was interested and paid attention to the conversation. For the next few days, we reminded him of the "rule." He adhered to the rule and stopped pulling his hair out.

Elizabeth: One of the most disturbing parts of autism for me is when my children engage in self-injurious behavior or self-abuse. I think one reason is that the label "self-injurious" heightens the seriousness of this behavior. Self-injurious is when someone causes harm or injury to themselves, so we automatically think of individuals who cut themselves or endanger their lives due to desperate acts for needed attention or to alleviate other personal pain. Looking at it that way causes us such undue stress and helplessness as parents. But with our children, that is not the case. Our children are not actually trying to hurt themselves. We need to look at their intentions, which may include filling sensory needs, rituals, misinterpretation of stimuli, and comfort. To watch my young daughter pound her head against the glass patio door is excruciating. To see her pick at just a pinprick scratch and dig at it until it was the size of a nickel is horrible. Watching Nathan repeatedly peel off the skin around his fingers and toes and leaving them raw is almost unbearable. I think they all have bitten themselves. We are still working with Chase. He will bite himself if he is incredibly overstimulated.

We also have had a hair-pulling issue. Nicole would find whatever she could to tangle in her hair and pull it out. A toothbrush was her most common weapon of choice, but the most dangerous were strings, ropes, and even hair ribbons. Nothing could be over seven inches long in our home. She would wrap anything she can get her hands on around her neck and then squeeze, enjoying the pressure.

But that is the key. She enjoys it. She is not trying to injure herself. Once I began to understand that, I could help her develop different ways to fill that need. I sought things that help to provide for her needs but in safer ways. And never, ever did I try to just remove a behavior. I would always give her a replacement behavior. Always. The consequence of leaving children unfulfilled encourages them to seek out their own replacement behavior, usually of increased intensity.

Like most behaviors of autism, if we can understand the reason (or at least have a best guess), we can help our children to develop strategies for coping or filling needs. I am no longer afraid of self-injurious behaviors. My children don't have deep-rooted emotional issues attached to their behaviors that I must counsel them in. For those families, my heart goes out to them, and I wish them the best.

Dr. B: Children with ASD tend to rely on rules and routine patterns to make their environment seem more predictable, and therefore seem safer. These rules might be the rules for any given situation they find themselves in or rules they themselves have invented for any situation. They seem to take comfort in rules and insist on the enforcement of all rules. Teenagers on the spectrum have described that rules give them a sense of order and help them to feel anchored. This feeling of security is lost if the rule is not specific enough and becomes a source of conflict. Elise, a camp counselor at a summer camp for children with autism, tells us of a sign in the mess hall at dinner. The sign read, "Please take just one cookie." Elise noticed one evening Calvin had three cookies after dinner. She approached the subject in a nonthreatening manner and told him the rule is that each person is only to take one cookie. He said he knew the rule and had followed the rule. When she asked him how it happens that he had three cookies he patiently explained to her he had gone up to the dessert table three separate times. Each time he had just taken one cookie, as the sign said. He explained to her the sign did not say "and then do not come back."

Parents and educators can use the rule-governed behavior to our best advantage. Ethan was a gregarious teenager who greeted people happily in the morning.

However, he perseverated on the routine of greeting and continued to greet the same people all day long with the same social salutations of the morning. Each time during the day, when his eyes landed on a person, he greeted them anew, disrupting the class. We set up a "rule" that he should only greet each teacher and student the first time he sees them every day. To make that easier, when Ethan greeted a person each day, they would stick a colored paper dot on their shirt collar. This was a visual reminder to Ethan that he had already said, "Good morning, how are you?" to that person on that day, and it was not appropriate to ask them again. When we set a rule, it must be clear and define the expectation. Visual aids are helpful. For the early learner, this may be in the form of a visual schedule. For the more advanced child, the rule may be written and posted. If the rule is complex, it needs to be broken down into the requisite steps. We find it more successful to state the rule in the positive, such as "walk," rather than in the negative, "don't run." It seems to be a more successful approach to tell the child what we *do* want them to do rather than what we *don't* want them to do.

One technique we use for teaching rules is a rehearsal of the social rules. We actually set up scenarios and practice social strategies such as how to join a conversation. An aspect of the rule-governed behavior that makes life difficult for family members is that the child with autism may tend to create his own rules and expect others to follow the rules or rituals he has made up. Even though it may be a complicated ritual connected to a daily activity, the family may allow it and even go along with it because it is easier than dealing with the meltdown that will ensue if it is not followed. Families describe tiptoeing around a whole regime of rules imposed upon the household by the child with autism because it simply is not worth the fight. They tell of child imposed rules such as, "No leaving the house through the garage," "No screaming sound when you sneeze," "Pizza every Friday and meatloaf on Wednesday," "No eating breakfast food at supper," and "No teeth touching the fork."

Mrs. Luck: I talked with a mom who never moves the furniture in her house because when she does, her son has a behavior breakdown that lasts for three weeks. Heaven forbid that she ever buy a *new* chair! She also never has company in the house because it upsets the boy too much and just isn't worth the emotional toll it takes on the whole family. When friends or family come from out of state, she meets them at a local restaurant to avoid the meltdown. I know another family who can never eat sandwiches at dinner time, just at lunch, and another whose son insists they have a set menu for each day of the week. A mother last week described to me that her son will never wear clothing a sibling has worn, or from a yard sale even after it is washed multiple times. These are examples of rules made up by the child and imposed not only on him but on the other family members.

Mrs. Nic: One challenge is that in reality different situations have different rules. These kids tend to feel a rule is more concrete and should not change with the situation. When children with autism are mainstreamed into regular education classes, they have a hard time understanding that there may be different rules in the regular education class. Whereas the special education class may have had five students enrolled in it, the regular education class may have closer to thirty, so the regular education teacher needs to set different, more formal rules. Alex, who was mainstreamed for about half the day, was designated as the "line leader" in the special education room one day. When he came to the regular education second grade, he started shoving others aside, insisting it was his day to be the line leader. He could not be convinced that since there were twenty-seven children in the second grade, his turn to be line leader was every twenty-seventh day. His turn to be line leader in his special education classroom was every five days.

Mrs. Luck: It is important to kids with autism to be rule followers. If you have a class rule, they will follow it and feel it is their duty and responsibility to make everyone, including you, follow that rule. Sometimes, rules carry over from school to home. I taught Charlie in a self-contained classroom. The rule at school was: you refer to a teacher as Miss. We had Ms. Nora, Ms. Barbie, and Ms. Jan. His mother called school and said, "I think it is cute when he calls me Ms. Mommy, but his dad doesn't appreciate it when Charlie calls him Ms. Daddy."

I had a fifth-grade Asperger's student who came to speech on Thursdays at 9:00 and left to go to PE at 9:30. One day, during speech, we had a practice lockdown drill. Everything was fine until 9:30.

"Mrs. Luck, it is 9:30, and I go to PE at 9:30."

"Yes, I know, but we are having a special practice, so we will know what to do in case there is an emergency."

"Is there an emergency?"

"No, this is just a practice."

"Then I'm going to PE."

This conversation was repeated every three minutes until I said, "The rule is you go to PE on Thursdays at 9:30 unless we are having a special emergency practice, an assembly, or anything else your teacher, the principal, or I tell you about."

"Okay, tell me when I can go to PE."

Some teachers say, "This is usually our schedule, and I will tell you if we are having something different today." Sometimes a quiet two-minute warning helps with transitioning from one activity to another.

The child on the spectrum gets frustrated if the rules are not clear. One of our children kept getting in trouble in music class. I asked him, "What can Mrs. Music Teacher do to help you do better in music?" He simply explained, "She can tell me how many warnings she is going to give me before she gets mad. Sometimes, it's two, and sometimes, it's four. I don't know when I really need to stop talking." I personally think his request is fair and logical. After all, why should he get in trouble because she is not consistent in her expectations? So the teachers had discussed this and agreed to define the limits for him. The student went to music the next time. Mrs. Music Teacher said, "I will give you two warnings, and then I will move you from your friends. You will not be able to move back during this class period." Immediately, the student started talking, and the teacher looked at him. Several minutes later, the student started talking again, and the teacher looked at him. The student was quiet and on task for the rest of the class. Everyone was happy.

Dr. B: Besides the strong desire for consistent rules, children on the spectrum characteristically show extreme resistance to change of any kind. Strong adherence to routine is helpful as a coping mechanism for their everyday life. The need for sameness has been described as a reaction to the processing of an unexpected stimulus. The difficulty in accepting change in routine makes some things particularly difficult, such as travel. Military families or others who must move often describe trauma at each move. Jaxon's mom was anticipating a cross-country move and told me she expected it will take him at least six months to adjust. When I was watching the TV coverage of the wildfires in California, the news station did a story about a family that had lost their home and all their belongings. One child in the family was a thirteen year-old-boy with autism. Although I felt sad for all of the people who lost their homes, my heart particularly went out to this family, knowing how stressful this type of change would be for a child on the autism spectrum. All his toys, all his clothing, his home, and the family belongings would all need to be replaced. I can't even imagine how difficult this was for that family.

Mrs. Nic: In our school, the best teachers who have children with autism or Asperger's in their classes give notice of impending transitions, such as "In ten minutes, we will start circle time," followed by another notice at five and two minutes, and one minute. When it is time to change the activity, they announce the start of the new activity, and commence a backward count of, "Three, two, one. Okay, everyone please come to circle time."

Mrs. Luck: Another great strategy is the use of visual timers. The teacher can set the timer for any number of minutes. There is a visual signal that rotates showing the amount of time left on the timer.

Dr. B: Looking at each individual child in reference to all these differences and commonalities can give a good indication of the presence of autism or Asperger's. Elise, the counselor at Camp Encourage, explains red flags this way: "Children on the spectrum are each totally unique. They have vastly different abilities and personalities. However, they all have that similar intangible autism trait that makes me think, 'Aha! That's autism.'"

SECTION III

You Are Not Alone— Know Your Team Members

To succeed as a team is to hold all of the members accountable for their expertise.

—Mitchell Caplan,
CEO E*Trade Group Inc.

Educational Professionals

Dr. B: The most comprehensive and effective treatment for any person with autism requires a team of providers. The diagnostic and treatment path can get very complicated, especially since each child's need is different. There is not one "cookbook" answer to the people who will comprise your team. It falls to the parents to assemble an appropriate team of providers.

When you to choose to involve your child in formal education, the relationship between the student and the teacher becomes of paramount importance. Whether the teacher comes to your home or your child attends an educational facility, the educator begins to assert a strong influence on the student's life.

Over the years, I have worked with quite a variety of teachers. Some had no more than a high school education, while others had advanced degrees in education. Some were old, and some were young. Personalities and teaching styles vary. When the time came for me to be in a position to hire teachers and to formally evaluate the staff, I began to search for what factors were critical in determining teacher excellence for children with special needs. Why were some teachers so successful and "tuned in" to the world of autism? My realization was that some teachers just "get it" while others never do. For those who get it, I feel strong admiration. For those do not, I feel sympathy. To be in this type of teaching position and not get it must be miserable. It is interesting that the ability to get it does not seem to be tied to education level or experience, although both of those factors can enhance the teacher's performance.

The same is true for teacher aides or assistants. These paraprofessionals are an important part of the classroom equation and serve as an extension of the teacher. Paras may work directly with students or they may spend time doing clerical activities, thereby allowing the teacher more time to teach.

Mrs. Nic: I read an article just this week that was intended to encourage teachers to accept the challenge of working with children with autism. The article states that there is *no difference* in teaching typical children compared to teaching children with autism. The author of that article is an example of someone who "doesn't get it." Any teacher who follows that philosophy of teaching special needs children is doing a great disservice to the children as well as to herself.

Dr. B: In a dissertation conducted at the University of Louisville, Wilkerson studied teacher attitudes toward the inclusion of students with autism into regular education classrooms.[13] In this study nearly all regular education teachers reported that they were not appropriately trained to work with students on the spectrum. Shockingly, over half of the special education teachers stated that they were not adequately trained to work with students with autism. In general, the teachers reported a lack of formal training on the topic of autism.

Although the teachers in that study felt that educating children with autism should be a team effort between special education teachers and regular education teachers, the majority of them felt that the best way to do that was through a consult model. They supported keeping autistic students in separate classrooms to better meet their needs.

I sat in an IEP meeting with a teacher who would be getting a student with ASD mainstreamed into her class of typical students. Although the child was nonverbal and low functioning, he was being mainstreamed into her class for socialization with age-matched peers. The teacher announced to the parent in this IEP meeting, "You know *all* autistic children are really geniuses." At that point, she lost credibility with those at the table who have taken the time and effort to educate themselves on the topic of autism.

In contrast, at another IEP meeting, I read a section of the IEP form that asks for the teacher to list the child's strengths. This is a crucial bit of information as it helps the team decide how to teach this child. The teacher who filled out the form had listed the child's only strength as "His body temperature is 98.6." If that is the only positive thing your child's teacher can see in your child, I'd suggest changing educational providers.

On the other hand, I have worked with many teachers who have a strong knowledge base and a talent for individualizing programming to meet each child's special needs. They know the children and are willing to put in a monumental effort to teach each child in the style that the child learns best. These teachers are caring, dedicated, and work long, hard hours to provide for your child.

Shelli: I couldn't wait to get to this section because to me it is an area that exudes hope.

I struggled with letting go of Joshuah at three years of age to send him to school on a bus with people who we didn't know. I did not trust that they would be able to handle my son. He was more than a handful. I was afraid they would take their eyes off him, and I would never see him again. I understood my son. He wasn't able to use words to explain his thoughts or wants and needs, but I could "read his mind." I knew my son's thoughts at the minute they entered his mind. I had "super mom powers." After First Steps, a program at the local public school was the next step in getting the assistance I would need to follow through with his early childhood education, and I was terrified. I held off sending him for almost a year. That year, we had none of the therapy that was so desperately needed. During that time, I had talked with the insurance companies in an effort to get him into a program that would offer the therapies he needed. Insurance wouldn't cover the programs we were looking at. So I let go of my "super mom" complex and turned loose. I toured the school, met the teachers and the staff, and they were wonderful. Joshuah didn't stress them out like I thought he would. I have to say by our second year of early childhood I was hooked. I had a great relationship with the staff. We worked together as a team.

During Joshuah's second year of school, his sister, Israyel, joined him. She was only three, but because of the relationship I had established with the school, I felt totally comfortable with the staff and chose to send my sweet little girl to school with no hesitation. They were both in the same class, and this was an added comfort. Knowing the people who are working with your child is so important. My advice is for you to make the extra effort to reach out and cement that relationship. Teachers are there to help you, and together, you can achieve the goals that have been set for your child. Teachers really are amazing people. They come up with such creative ways to break down so many of those obstacles our precious kids face daily.

Dr. B: We had a young girl named Kelsey who was difficult to motivate. She was content to be noncompliant and refused do the tasks that the teacher, Ms. White, had designed for her. Kelsey's mom was discussing the behavior with Ms. White. The mom felt it would be better to just let Kelsey sit and watch, to ask nothing of her, so as not to upset her. Ms. White refused to let Kelsey take such an easy way out and demanded the best out of Kelsey. Kelsey's mom became upset and said to Ms. White, "You don't *love* Kelsey, or you wouldn't push her so hard!" Ms. White replied, "It's *your* job to *love* her. It's *my* job to *teach* her."

Elizabeth: We have had some great teachers. Most of them really try. There is one thing I want teachers to know though: the deal breaker. The relationship crusher is saying to parents, "Well, he doesn't do that here. We don't see that behavior at school." It is probably meant to be helpful: to highlight that there are different stressors in different environments. Even if you are truly trying to isolate a trigger, don't say it. The strongest of parents' knees will buckle. Some will be willing to bite their tongues. When we hear this, it feels like the school is trying to blame the home, that the teacher and staff are better at this than the parents. Please know this hurts. There are many things to consider when looking at behaviors at home verses school. It is comparing apples to oranges. I have heard it too many times. When it bothers me, I remind them I prepare my child to have a good day at school, and I would like to take credit for some of that behavior. Sometimes, by the time he gets home after holding it together for his education, he is done. That is okay with me. But most often, I take a deep breath and move on, realizing it is not meant to judge me.

Dr. B: An important part of the teacher's responsibility is to coordinate with other educational professionals involved in the child's program. One of those is the diagnostician. The role of the educational diagnostician will vary state to state. Even the title may be different depending on the geographical area. In general, the duties of the diagnostician include, but are not limited to, administering and interpreting educational tests, providing behavior management recommendations for both home and school, and consulting with teachers and parents. The educational diagnostician most often has previous experience as a classroom teacher. This same role may be filled by an ABA consultant in some facilities.

The ABA consultant will be either certified as a BCBA (board certified behavior analyst) or a BCaBA (board certified assistant behavior analyst). This is a fairly new discipline, with the certification boards established in 1998. The consultant may be an employee of the facility where your child goes for services or may be a private contractor. The BCaBA works under the supervision of a BCBA. This person will conduct behavioral assessments and make recommendations for your child.

You will see and hear of people who refer to themselves as an ABA therapist or a behavior consultant. These titles mean nothing. Always ask the person if they are board certified and ask them to show you their behavior analyst certificate. I have had some job applicants tell me they are ABA therapists, then try to talk circles around the fact that they are not board certified. Check out the credentials fully. You can review your state's behavior analyst certification board online registries to be sure the therapist is listed.

The speech-language pathologist (SLP) is another crucial member of your team. To be nationally certified (CCC or Certificate of Clinical Competence) by the American Speech-Language-Hearing Association (ASHA), she will have at least a master's degree in communication sciences and disorders. The labels "speech therapist" and "speech clinician" may also be used. The SLP assesses deficits in various areas of speech, language, and cognitive-communication and works with the client to improve these skills. In most cases, she will be a valued resource for you. Seek out one with a special interest in this population. Truthfully, a large number of SLPs are actually afraid of working with this demographic because they just don't know what to do to help. As in many other fields, the training has changed extensively over the years. Interestingly enough, speech pathologists trained in the 1960s and 1970s were given a strong base in the methods that have now come back into vogue. The techniques seen as the best approach in many colleges during those decades are those now being used successfully in ABA therapy. As time went on, different practices came into favor in remediation of speech and language, so university training from the 1980s to the millennium often had a different emphasis. Unfortunately for the field of language therapy, many of the therapists trained in the 60s and 70s have now retired or soon will. In those days, colleges had strong bachelor degree programs and graduated speech therapists that are still practicing in some places. These bachelor level therapists with lifelong experience are often very strong, highly skilled in dealing with children with special needs. Don't count them out. The older therapist nearing retirement and the new graduates will likely have strong backgrounds in the remediation of the language difficulties of children on the spectrum. Those who were educated in the in-between years will be comfortable with this population if they have developed their knowledge and taken on cases that enhance their understanding. Talk to the SLP you are considering working with. Look past the degrees and diplomas on the wall. Observe her at work with the child. Your heart will tell you if she "gets it."

Occupational therapists work on sensory integration, coordination, fine motor skills, and self-help. They deal with many practical areas of daily life such as feeding and dressing.

Shelli: I have deep respect for OTs. Often, when dealing with pediatricians on sensory issues, I would have rather talked with an OT. Occupational therapists were often able to look at my son and say, "I bet this is why he is doing this," tell me what to do, and it worked. I would call the pediatrician, and he would end up telling me my kid was just having an "off day." We all have bad days, right? But in my gut, I would know there was something else amiss. Don't get me wrong, physicians are an important part of your team, but when they can't give you an answer about your child's sensory needs, talk to an OT.

Dr. B: Music therapy is another accepted mental health profession, which has a connection to autism. A professional music therapist holds a bachelor's degree or higher in music therapy. Music therapists should be board certified. After assessing the strengths and needs of each child, the therapist provides the indicated treatment including creating, singing, moving to, and/or listening to music. I have to confess that until I saw music therapy in action, I did not have total appreciation for its educational value. I have become a convert as I have seen children on the spectrum show a heightened interest and response to music. It is an excellent therapeutic tool. Music can actually stimulate cognitive activity and can be a bridge to communication for children with ASD.

Mrs. Nic: Think about how you learned your ABCs. You likely learned to sing them. Commercials use music and song to imbed telephone numbers and product recognition into our minds. In that same way, the music therapist can teach concepts at the child's cognitive level.

Medical Professionals

Shelli: Finding the right physician for your child is so important. Doctor's offices have often been a point of stress for my kids. The children don't know what to expect. Some places just push you in and out so fast that the kids don't know what hit them. Getting on the phone and talking with the physician beforehand can be really helpful. Remember, you want someone who is going to be a team player, not another person who doesn't understand how to work with your child. Unfortunately, not all physicians are "autism savvy." I suggest asking questions like "Do you have other patients with autism?" Then, I watch them interact with my kids on our first visits. Are they gentle? Did they give my child a chance to feel comfortable with them while they were in the room with us? I also ask this question that is helpful for us: When is the slowest time of the day for you? I don't want to come and sit for hours in a waiting room with my kids when the room is crowded and loud. That just gets them worked up. Ask if the staff is willing to let you go into a room in the back while you wait. Before the appointment, I always write down the information the doctors will need, so when we go in, I can just hand it to the nurse ahead of time. That way, when the doctor comes in, she already knows the details, and we can get in and out much faster. Remember, we are working together as a team. I want to help them out because I want their help. It is a two-way street.

Dr. B: Some primary care physicians are not confident in their knowledge of autism. A study of over 3,000 pediatricians and family practice doctors concluded that in general these primary care physicians reported a self-perceived lack of skills dealing with this population. They reported that they wanted further education on the topic.[14]

Mrs. Nic: Another good plan is to call ahead to make sure the doctor is running on time. If not, ask how far delayed the appointments are. If you get an unexpected delay when you get to the doctor's office, take your child and go wait in your car rather than the reception area. The office staff can call you on your cell phone when the doctor is ready to see you. Be sure to bring toys or items to entertain your child during the wait.

Some parents practice the doctor visit using a toy doctor kit. Do whatever you can to limit sensory overload and to reduce the factor of surprise.

Mrs. Luck: Autism Speaks has partnered with Colgate, Philips, and Sonicare to produce a quick and easy guide for dentists, which will educate them in working with children on the spectrum.[15] It is available online and contains very practical suggestions. If your dentist really wants to work with special needs children, he will be receptive to looking at this tool and implementing the suggestions. Don't be shy about offering it to your dental staff!

Dr. B: Because of the child's lack of consistent responses to sounds, one of the first medical professionals you see may be an audiologist. Hearing screenings might be unsuccessful because behavioral difficulties may interfere with the results. Look around for an audiologist who has an interest in working with special needs children. Let him know what things are reinforcing to your child, and he can use those rewards to facilitate the evaluation. You can assure a smoother visit by having your child practice the motor movements he will need to make in order to signal that he hears the stimulus tones. Talk to the audiologist before the visit, and he will guide you in this practice.

Some of the best audiological screening I have seen for special needs children has been done by our local university hearing clinic. The audiology students came to our school and spent time getting to know each child before the actual screening day. They learned how to communicate with each child and let the child get comfortable with them. In some cases, the testers asked the parents to bring the child to the university hearing clinic to make use of more specialized equipment needed to assess the child's hearing.

Another critical member of your support team is your neurologist. Neurologists specialize in problems associated with the nervous system, especially the brain, spinal cord, muscles, and nerves. You may come into contact with the neurologist when seeking a diagnosis or in follow-up treatments. If your child has neurological co-morbidities or if he has lost abilities he previously had, you will likely get connected with this specialist.

Many times, the involvement of the neurologist is based on a child's seizures or ADHD.

Since your pediatrician is the medical person you will depend on as your base for references, you should contact your pediatrician if your child's behavior begins to change in any negative way. If your child starts to experience episodes of rage or out of control behavior or if you begin to notice self-injurious behavior, you should call the pediatrician who knows your child. Together, you can then decide if further referral is warranted or if other testing needs to be conducted. If your child is referred to a therapist, you will find a variety of professionals who provide this service.

Clinical social workers (CSWs) are mental health professionals who have master's degrees in social work and are licensed to practice psychotherapy. CSWs cannot prescribe drugs, so they refer their patients to psychiatrists if there is a need to evaluate for medication.

Elizabeth: Another team member similar to the CSW could be your caseworker. We have had many caseworkers. I have had some who are very involved and others who just did the minimal paperwork needed. Some parents have the misconception about caseworkers that they will help you find all the resources your child needs. They will help you with the ones they know about and if you bring things to their attention, they may help follow through. This may possibly include help finding funding sources. But as parents, we cannot rely on our caseworkers to give us all the answers. They are there to help facilitate things. As your child gets older and may need more services, it will be important to have an involved caseworker because funding of services often has to go through them. Our current caseworker asks to attend IEP meetings so she can stay informed about the boys' progress.

Dr. B: Psychologists explore different mind-sets and emotional problems such as self-harming, depression, etc. Their training is based on human behavior. A psychologist is a non-medical health-care professional who has a master's degree or doctorate in psychology and treats people using therapeutic methods. They do not normally prescribe medications, although some states allow limited writing of prescriptions. If you are looking for pharmaceuticals, you could choose to go to a psychiatrist.

A psychiatrist is able to prescribe medication in addition to doing counseling. A psychiatrist is a licensed medical doctor who specializes in abnormalities of the mind (not the brain, that's a neurologist). You may find the psychiatrist's fees are higher than the charges of a social worker or a psychologist.

Mrs. Luck: Parents often ask at what point they should seek professional help for the behaviors. I think they should be looking for negative changes in the child's behaviors. Definitely seek help if your child seems out of control, is in danger of hurting himself or others, or goes into a state of rage.

Mrs. Nic: If the child's behavior scares you in any way, ask for help. If you have any doubt, the pediatrician can help you make this judgment. Along with taking a written list of concerns to your appointment, some parents find it helpful to take a videotape of the behavior that concerns you. That way, the professionals can see exactly what you are dealing with.

Community

Dr. B: Lately, I have been reading about lawsuits filed by people who want a child with ASD in the neighborhood to be legally confined to his own house and yard. One person blogging online was worried that a four-year-old neighbor with autism might get his hands on a firearm and come out shooting. I have even seen websites that give advice on how to get families evicted from your condominium association because their child with autism is too noisy.

In contrast, other communities are offering special activities for families who are dealing with autism, such as "sensory night" at the local movies. The theater provides a welcoming atmosphere with lower volume and a theater that isn't so dark. In these special showings, children are not restricted from verbal outbursts. The other people in the audience understand and are not judgmental. Some cities have "sensory night" at the local inflatable bounce house, or special events at the city parks.

Shelli: Autism Speaks distributes an emergency packet parents can give to their neighbors.[16] The information in the packet explains autism and what to do if you see this child out alone in the neighborhood. You can include your phone number and a picture of your child, so he is easily recognized. I got the packet, and it has come in handy. I have only given the packet to the people who I know in the neighborhood, which are about five families. Josh got out without me knowing it once. I got a phone call from a neighbor telling me that Joshuah was by their house, and they had him contained in their car. I was able to go get him without any judgment from them, and Josh wasn't harmed.

My husband and I have two children with autism, but we are not the only ones affected by it. Grandparents now have grandkids with autism; aunts and uncles now have nieces and nephews with autism. If you are a relative, I know that these are not your own children, but they are a part of your family. Take time to educate yourself. Be involved in their schools, take them to the park for the evening, take them to McDonald's, and play with them. They need you just as much as they need their parents. Family is so important to this process. Through this experience, I have come to understand the value of family. You need them.

Grandparents who are willing to be there for you and help you out are so needed. Grandparents, if you're wondering "What can I do?" here it is: be there to listen. Sometimes, it helps the mom and dad to have someone who loves them enough to just listen. So step up. Set aside your ideas of normalcy and love these children unconditionally. Sometimes, it is nice for the parents to get away, even for a short break. Sleep is difficult at times. Knowing that I can call my mom, dad, or my in-laws has been such a blessing to me. They come over and let me sleep for a few hours. I have been able to carry on with life with a little more clarity when someone has been able to step up in my place for a while.

Elizabeth: Along with relatives, your friends are a crucial support system. Because we are in the same place at the same time, friendships naturally develop with other parents of children with autism. We tend to work on projects together. Often families of children with so many needs bond during activities they are participating in together. Kind of like the old saying regarding two birds with one stone. Our time is so consumed by activities and therapeutic endeavors that the only time we have to be social is in the waiting room or sitting on the sidelines at the Miracle Field as a "buddy" takes our place for that hour. That is commonly the progression I see.

But there is another piece to that. It is important to have a variety of friends. Each has her own personality and enriches our lives in different ways. I have found sometimes it is difficult to get to know others. What is important and on my mind is not the same for a person who doesn't have a child with special needs. While their conversations may center upon the amount of time spent helping their child prepare for spelling tests and the after school clubs, we talk about preparing for IEPs or the substitute para who aided in our child's meltdown. We listen to stories about their child's first goal, while dying to tell someone that our seven-year-old finally used the toilet. So we don't. We keep quiet and wait for someone who gets it. I have found when I talk about our daily activities, I am given compassion and pity in return. That is not what I am looking for in a friend. My child may need a buddy to play on his ball team and may need to use his iPad to tell me he wants to eat. That is my life. My miracle-filled incredible life. I want friends who will enjoy the journey with me, laugh at sensory issues, cry about setbacks, lift my spirits when I just think I can't go another day, and celebrate with me when my ten-year-old finally says "I love you" unprompted. That is why we find each other.

Dr. B: Church presents its own special set of challenges. It is often a setting with large crowds of people and, depending on the church, sometimes loud noises. Ideally, we will educate the church members about our children and do some preparation to help the church members accept the child as well as help the child adjust to the church situation. I hear many parents describe taking turns going to church while their partner stays home with the kids. Others describe dropping out of church for the years they are raising the child.

Mrs. Nic: I spent some time with Jane, a mom with three preschoolers on the spectrum. She was distraught and searching for answers to her dilemma about her church. She had attended this small church literally all her life—had grown up in that congregation. She just could not imagine ever changing churches. As she had children, her feelings began to change. She was told she could not leave her children in the nursery unless she and her husband stayed with them. This tiny country church did not have the advantage of video streaming to the nursery as some churches have. So the family of five would get all dressed up, go to church, and all sit in the nursery. She tried to keep a pleasant attitude and model and teach the staff during her visits to the nursery. The nursery was crowded, understaffed, smelled of dirty diapers in the trash, and there were multiple teachers giving directions. Children were yelling as teachers were trying to round them up to go to the tables for lessons or crafts. Other children were crying for their moms. She noticed as the teachers began to feel out of control, they would get louder and stricter. This spiraling scenario would set her children off into a meltdown. When music was introduced, it would be played at an abnormally high volume to be heard above the chaos. Church soon became the last place her children wanted to be.

She was dismayed because no one seemed to want to take the time to actually get to know her children. The nursery workers were judgmental about her children's behaviors. They asked her weekly why her children were not yet potty trained and she overheard teachers saying they did not want her preschoolers in their class because they were not about to change diapers. She heard them say they were afraid her children would scare the other children. She asked to set up a buddy system and was told it would be a liability for the church. She asked for a quiet room for families to retreat to when needed but was told all those empty rooms might be needed for something else one day. She would routinely leave in the middle of services in tears.

Her heart was broken when the ladies from the church would bring her books about how to be a better parent. I lost track of Jane for about a year, and the next time I saw her, she happily told me she had made the brave move and found a church where her whole family is accepted.

Elizabeth: Many families feel they cannot attend church. Time and time again, I hear families are made to feel bad and are even asked to leave because of the distraction of their family member's behaviors. My heart goes out to those families. It is very important and only fair that families who are living with disabilities receive spiritual edification. There are many churches who try to fill this void for parents by offering special classes and special needs ministries.

There are many technical aspects we could talk about for helping churches set up classes and train teachers. But that is a larger movement and not a quick answer to get our families who want to attend church to return. So often, it must fall on the families. Church is a very personal and up-close experience. Often, we think the stares are due to judgment. If there is one place they are not, it is at church. I have often misinterpreted the looks and avoidance as judgment. Luckily, I have grown a pretty thick skin and am confident in what I am doing. But it was still there, keeping me from forming relationships and participating fully in our church organization. Then seemingly out of nowhere, someone would approach me and tell me what a wonderful job I was doing or talk about how they love to watch my children attend. But it wasn't out of nowhere. It built week after week as our family continued to attend meetings, usually late, often eating, and always loud. What I didn't see was that the stares were of understanding and admiration. The lack of conversation was due to not knowing what to say. The lack of appropriate responses was due to unfamiliarity and inexperience with children who have special needs. They knew what to do if a child fell in the hallway, escaped from the nursery, or tore a hymn book. But they didn't know how to help if my child was having a meltdown or yelling during the prayer. So they sat, waited, and watched. What I didn't know is that they were learning. Watching me. It didn't happen overnight. It took time. Now as we attend church people kneel to be eye level with the boys, wait patiently for responses, and tell them how happy they are to see them.

I think we are some of the lucky ones. Is it because my expectations are lower on what I want my church to provide? Probably. Is it right? I don't know. I watch my friends go from church to church, seeking a program that will teach their children principles of religion. Often, they are frustrated in their quest. I see others deciding on a religion by what it offers their child, not necessarily filling their own beliefs or needs. This is often a big trial families face. Even today, as I sat in the hall, I wondered if it would have been better just to stay home. Then when classes were over and yet another family let Nathan hold their baby (with assistance) and he let out his happy sounds, I knew we were in the right place.

Dr. B: I have outlined some suggestions for churches to create a happy situation for families of special needs children.

A good start is to set up a buddy system. Anyone can be a buddy. In some places, kids in the youth group can volunteer. Ask a young person in the class to be a buddy, just to be a friend. It is a good learning experience for the volunteer and works toward the mission of the church.

Your family can often tap into the local agencies that will come to churches and do training and educating on autism. The agency can customize the training to your specific child's needs. They can even do training with the others in the class to help them better understand the child who has a diagnosis of autism. After such training, the other children are better able to understand when the child dealing with autism is having meltdowns or needs modifications in the rules. Adjustments can be made easier when everyone has a general knowledge and understanding of autism. This is easy, and it is free.

Reserve a room for calm downtime. This provides a chance for a child who has escalated to meltdown mode a place to calm down. I envision a nursery like room not overly decorated or stimulating.

Some children are just not able to handle large classrooms. It is okay for these kids to be in a separate room if it means success for the whole family.

Have a form available for families that asks about likes and dislikes, triggers, and other helpful things like allergies. Maybe include an emergency number. Mom or Dad in the sanctuary can be silently buzzed on their cell phones if there is an issue.

Plan ahead. Spend time outside of class getting to know the child. Work with these families by putting together picture schedules and social stories to help the class move more smoothly.

It is important to build trust between teacher and child. Keep open communication between the teacher and parents. If you are the teacher, try really hard to think, "If this were my child, what would my expectation and hope be?" Open your heart, and do whatever you can to help these families seeking time to worship. Parents love it when they are able to drop their kids off and just be free to leave and not worry if the people who are in charge are going to do their very best with them. No worries. It is a tremendous gift a congregation can give. Most importantly, the church members need to understand that children with autism are different but not less.

Many parents find that lifeline in a support group they have joined. Parental support groups may be face-to-face groups that meet together, but there is also a growing movement of online support systems for parents. There are many different types of autism support groups, and their activities vary, depending on the group's focus and goals. Some are very general and have members representing the full range of the spectrum. Others are specific and focus on a given functional level, a given sex or age, or a given program. Some schools organize their own parent support groups.

In a support group, you can expect to meet others who are facing the same challenges you are. Members of a group provide mutual support and share information. A group may be more formal and arrange for speakers on topics of interest. Families use group time to set up play dates or arrange to trade babysitting. In support groups, families find a sense of community and mutual understanding.

The other parents in your support groups, whether formal or informal gatherings, will pick you up when you need it. They validate your feelings because they share the struggles and the joys. You will pool your resources and share information. They are nonjudgmental because they are the ones who really, really get it.

The Parents' Role

Shelli: The parents' role is very important. You are the voice for your children. You are the first line of safety for them. You know what they are capable of and you are going to be the driving force that will either make or break your child's chances for success. You are an advocate. Educate yourself in all things autism. Find out what is out there. Look for resources. They are out there, but you have to look for them. As a parent, you are totally involved in your child's treatments, daily schedules, and daily stresses that are placed on the caretaker. It can be physically, mentally, and emotionally draining.

Elizabeth: I am an autism advocate and mother with powerful friends. I know how to get things done. Finding the energy to actually do it, though, is my lifelong pursuit. While searching for that energy I have managed to speak to politicians, fund-raise, plan conferences, be on various boards serving autism families, write and blog, including an article in *Autism Asperger's Digest*. I have been a member of the Missouri Parent Advisory Committee on Autism and have spent time in front of the camera and in the newspaper sharing our family's story to promote autism awareness.

Dr. B: Depending on what issues your child is facing at different points, be prepared to make changes to your team. The child's challenges will not remain stagnant but will evolve with time, and you need to have team members waiting in the wings ready to step in when needed.

SECTION IV

Interventions

Hope doesn't come from calculating whether the good news is winning out over the bad. It's simply a choice to take action.

—Anna Lappe

Behavioral Interventions

Dr. B: Muse Watson described how he felt as he and his wife searched for autism treatments. He said it felt like "two blind hogs rooting for acorns." Interventions for autism include educational, behavioral, and biomedical treatments. Although these interventions do not cure autism, they often bring about improvements. Each child is different and has different needs. With your team, you will tailor your program to your child. There are hundreds of purported treatments for autism. We will discuss the methods that we find to be the most widely used, well-accepted methods.

Elizabeth: There are different techniques and programs available for working with a child with autism. Those involved in these programs are passionate and vocal about their work. Don't base your decision to be exclusive to their program on their passion but rather on what is best for your child and your family. By starting early, your child has the greatest potential. Be careful of doing intense work drills where no learning is going on.

Remember, learning can be as simple as learning to cope and comply. Anything your child is learning will need to be generalized (able to do in different situations) at some point. The time spent with your child in therapies, training, or teaching should be of a useful nature. There are some techniques that use reward systems or stimulus-response techniques. If you choose to go this route, please use properly trained therapists who know the complete program, not just the technique for getting a child to respond. The theories behind these techniques are usually much more involved than what we see on the surface and are vital to the success of that particular therapy or program.

The things you learn from the therapists can be incorporated into every activity you do with your children. It sounds hard and time-consuming, but it is less work than having an understimulated child with autism who is constantly biting or throwing tantrums.

Dr. B: Applied behavior analysis (ABA), also known as behavior modification, including the Lovaas method, is based on a science, which involves the application of basic behavioral principles (positive reinforcement, repetition, and prompting).[17] The vast majority of parents I have dealt with are believers in this technique. ABA, which requires strict adherence to data tracking, is found to be helpful in reducing problems such as self-injurious behaviors, transition, communication problems, and self-stimulatory behavior. An ABA program will be unique to your child and may include a variety of techniques. You may be surprised at how time intensive a strong program is. Your therapists will involve you in the therapy, and you will carry on the program throughout the hours that the child is not in formal therapy sessions.

Shelli: We have had a few ABA specialists in our home. There was one who we just loved. She worked a lot with getting Josh to make eye contact. She taught me about "reinforcers." If I want Joshuah to do something, he learns that he gets a reward when he complies with my request. This started out with toys. Joshuah's toy of choice was a Sesame Street toy with characters that would pop out and sing catchy little tunes. This later became Israyel's toy of choice too. I watched as Joshuah would grab my hand and put it on the toy called La, la, la, la Elmo's World when he wanted it to go. I would invite my family over just so they could see the miracles that were happening right in our home. Joshuah was learning how to tell us what he wanted rather throwing tantrums that required us to guess what he wanted. It was amazing. Through ABA, Joshuah learned he has to do something to get something.

I would have to say that to me, ABA is a must for kids on the spectrum. This method of teaching just seems to work.

Programs Based on Learning Theories

Dr. B: Other programs have foundations rooted in learning theory, including sensory integration, tactile, auditory, visual, or interdisciplinary programs. There are also some special therapies such as hippo-therapy (therapeutic horseback riding).

Elizabeth: Sensory therapy or sensory integration therapy is using play as a means to relay sensory pathways from the body to the brain. The more active your child is, the more he becomes tuned in to his body. As we work with our children, we are tempted to avoid certain activities because they are "just plain hard" or because of your child's resistance, behavior, physical hardships, and any number of reasons. The problem is, by avoiding certain activities, you may be depriving your child of sensations he needs to encourage better sensory pathways. An occupational therapist, especially one who is certified in sensory integration, can help individualize therapy techniques for your child. Remember that although therapists are a wonderful resource, they are normally only able to work with your child one to five hours a week. Learn from them and integrate that information into your own plan.

You will be using play to increase tolerance of stimuli, decrease tactile sensitivities, develop proper interaction with the environment, encourage balance and posture, help increase coordination, and improve motor planning. Overall, you will be helping your child become less sensitive to some stimuli and increase responses to others.

Dr. B: A recent study published in the online journal Research in Autism Spectrum Disorders links higher motor skills with increased social and communication skills in children with autism.[18] The author concludes that there is a link between poor motor skills and autism. There was also a correlation between development of good motor skills and a higher level of daily activities such as playing and talking.

Shelli: Children with ASD usually have difficulty receiving and responding to sensory stimuli and integrating information from the five senses. This is why it is important to obtain an assessment by an occupational or physical therapist with experience in autism. A "motor therapist" who is trained in sensory integration techniques can determine whether the child has difficulty in these areas. Suggestions made by the sensory integration therapist for individualized "sensory diet" activities should be incorporated frequently into the child's day, in all life settings, in order to maintain your child's level of comfort and cooperation. Having opportunities for regular, predictable sensory input may help the child during transitions. I find it also helps my children cope on their "off days" when nothing else seems to calm them.

The use of intensive sensory-motor activities for children who do not communicate verbally is strongly recommended. It seems successful with ASD children who fail to relate or have little interest in their environment. An intense SI program allows the child to eventually organize his world and be able to respond to other activities that can promote his communication and learning. I have seen serious behavioral problems resolved with adequate sensory input.

Teachers and parents should be aware children with ASD frequently have difficulty with motor planning (praxis). For example, even though their fine and gross motor functioning may otherwise be adequate, they may struggle with handwriting skills. If this is the case, the use of a computer to do schoolwork, both in the classroom and at home, should be viewed as a necessary prosthetic device, such as eyeglasses are for visually impaired persons. Many parents recommend the program Handwriting Without Tears, which has been successful in improving handwriting skills in ASD children.

Remember that teaching "skills" (whether occupational/physical therapy or speech) only in therapy sessions is inadequate—these techniques and supports must be integrated into everyday life. Persons with ASD frequently describe their difficulty with sensory hypersensitivities and/or dysfunctions throughout their lives, indicating that this problem is an almost universal aspect of the overall disability.

Dr. B: You may see children with autism wearing earphones at school or in the community. There are two types of earphones these children may be wearing. Children may struggle with auditory processing disorders. This means that they have trouble filtering out target sounds from background noise. For instance, they may tune into the sound of the air-conditioner running and not notice someone talking to them. For these students, the ear phones can be programmed to a microphone the teacher wears. This way, the background noise is blocked out, and the teacher's voice is amplified.

Other students are just hypersensitive to noise and wear noise reduction headphones in order to tolerate the environment. I have seen success using the noise-reducing earphones, both in school and in the community. Students who feel relief from the reduction of noise will eventually learn to come and ask for the headphones when they are overwhelmed by environmental noises.

There are also commercial listening programs, which basically use earphone systems to deliver specially filtered music. I have read individual endorsements online, but the few people I have talked to face-to-face who have tried them did not recommend those programs.

When a student uses equipment to maintain or improve function this is referred to as using assistive technology. Assistive technology falls into three basic categories: low tech, medium tech, and high tech. Typically, children with autism process visual information easier than they process auditory information. Any time we use assistive technology devices with these children, we are giving them information through their visual modalities, which is likely their strongest processing area. The products range from line drawings on a board to highly developed electronic devices. The important thing is that it must be individualized to your child following testing to determine the best system for his learning abilities and style.

An example of a successful program that focuses on visual supports is the Picture Exchange Communication System (PECS). Using PECS, nonverbal children can become successful in making their wants and needs known. The complexity of the symbols increases as the child masters the use of the symbols. PECS can be used in the school, the home, or even when they are out in the community.

Shelli: When Joshuah was exposed to the PECS (Picture Exchange Communication System), it opened a communication that helped him handle transitions and understand what was coming up next (scheduling). For the first time, Joshuah was showing signs that he was understanding what was expected of him. PECS helped with several negative behaviors we were dealing with at home and on outings in the community.

One of the most helpful therapeutic approaches is speech-language therapy. A speech-language pathologist evaluates a child's needs and strengths in several areas of language and designs a therapy program to improve the child's functional communication skills. Speech-language pathologists may work on developing receptive language, expressive language skills, or skills of social speech. One example of a technique for social reasoning is the social story.[19]

Mrs. Luck: A social story is an instrument designed by Carol Gray to help students think through social or behavioral situations to assure a better outcome the next time a similar situation arises. It is not telling a student what to do in a situation but helping them come to their own conclusion. Keep it simple and have the student sign the form when you are finished to help give him ownership of the decision. Don't make it a punishment, but a learning process.

A social autopsy is a way to break down a behavior into components so the student can better understand the situation and hopefully find a better solution next time. You can use social stories and autopsies with behaviors such as taking something that doesn't belong to him.

This is an example of a social story.

1. What happened? (Two to three short sentences in the student's own words. State facts, not opinions.)
   Child: I had a red car in my pocket. I told Mrs. Luck it was my car. It was Henry's car.
2. What was the error? (The student will need some help with this one.)
   Child: I said it was my car, and it was Henry's.
3. Who was hurt? (This could be physically or emotionally.)
   Child: Henry was feeling sad because he couldn't find his car.
4. What was the consequence?
   Child: I had to stay in for a recess. I can't play with any toys Henry brings to school.
5. What should happen next time? (This is the social story part.)

Child: I should give a car back after I play with it. I should not put something in my pocket that belongs to someone else even if I like it a lot and want to take it home.

The student and teacher or parent should both sign the form, and the student is given a copy.

Social stories can be as simple or complex as the student can relate to. It can help a student work through a situation that is causing him anxiety. You don't always have to fill out a form; sometimes, you can just talk him through the situation.

I had a student tell me he did not want to perform in the third-grade class program because he had stage fright and was afraid he would not be able to sing in front of strangers.

Autopsy (problem): inability to sing in front of strangers.

I asked him whom he would like to sing to, and he said he would like to sing to monkeys. I asked him how that could help the situation, and he said he could pretend the audience was full of monkeys. No more stage fright! His solution, not mine.

Dr. B: Most professionals today prefer the inter-disciplinary approach both in assessment and in treatment. In this approach, team members work together to provide the best programming for the child. This differs from a multidisciplinary approach, where there is a total team involved, but each is doing their own thing in their own way.

Some therapies are less traditional. One that gets rave reviews from most parents is therapeutic horseback riding. Therapeutic riding can be a fun way to incorporate OT, PT, and speech-language therapy into the session.

Elizabeth: I was so excited to take Nathan to his first hippotherapy session. I dreamed and prayed this therapy would touch him. I hoped the sadness and distance that is common in my young son would ease, at least for just a moment. It did but not for just a moment. It lasted well beyond the hour he spent with his new friend "Thunder." Nathan opened up his heart for this horse and his therapists. He let his happy sounds ring loud and free.

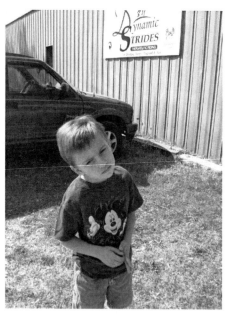

Nathan before therapy

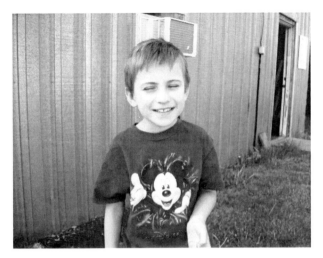

Nathan after therapy

Biomedical Interventions

Elizabeth: It seems to me when a parent or professional finds something that benefits a child on the spectrum, they run with it. They preach it to everyone who crosses their path. When our second child with autism started showing the early signs, everyone, including myself, thought, "He just needs to be taught sign language and then he will excel like his sister." Problem solved.

Hah, not quite. After working with him for a year, it was painfully obvious that sign language wasn't the key for him. In that experience, I learned what everyone says yet often fails to believe. What is preached is that every child is different and so is what works for them. If we truly believed this, then there wouldn't be that invisible line that separates families.

There is a great division between those who are passionate about biomedical treatments and those who believe strongly that traditional therapy is the only way to go. I have three children with autism, and successes have come about by a myriad of efforts. Each individual child is different and so is what works for them. As parents and professionals, we need to respect that difference and learn from others' experiences. Take what we need for our child and leave what can help another. Don't judge. Things that were once considered impossible are commonplace today. The time between the days of writing letters to the days of sending texts is not that long. What may seem odd today may be protocol in the future. As I have learned, there is no "one size fits all"; there's no single answer. Don't push other parents to agree with you. Respect differences in opinions. Don't let the one thing that should bond us become a dividing point.

The most common and least invasive type of biomedical intervention may be changing your child's diet. You may feel there are dietary concerns for your child. Maybe you have tried programs where you eliminate certain types of foods. This may be helpful, but you must not look for your child to simply be cured by removing the offending foods. If your child has dietary concerns, don't forget to include schooling, therapies, and your parent program.

While you may not be at the point where you are thinking you would like to remove all yeast products or all wheat products from your child's diet, you may wish to consider keeping a food diary. A food diary is basically writing down everything your child eats each day. As you do this, also record his behavior, including tantrums, outbursts, unresponsiveness, and lethargy. Do this chronologically. After charting this, begin to note extreme behaviors and what was eaten prior to the behavior. Do this for many weeks and see if a pattern develops. We were able to determine that apple juice was an almost instant trigger for tantrums with Nicole. It was explained to us that it poured too much sugar into her blood too quickly, and she went into overdrive. Later, I learned that the sugar in apples feeds yeast. Avoiding drinks with apple juice brought an immediate relief to some of her uncontrollable behavior.

When Nicole first began attending her second school, we spoke with her teachers and informed them of her sensitivity to apple juice. Together, we came to the conclusion that we would send a water bottle from home for her to use at snack time so she could avoid apple juice. As the first weeks went by, her teachers began to feel badly that they offered all of the other children juice while Nicole was served water. We allowed their request to give her juice while reminding them of possible consequences. That very afternoon, Nicole brought a note home asking us to send her water bottle to school.

As recommended by his early intervention team, at one point, we removed dairy from Nathan's diet. Quite often, experienced teachers and therapists are able to recognize the type of children who will respond to dietary intervention. After the first week of not being allowed any dairy, Nathan went through a sort of withdrawal. This is common. At this time, he also had much improved eye contact, which he had totally lost before beginning this diet. He also began to make speech sounds and basically gave us a glimmer of hope. The way he responded led his team to recommend we try a gluten-free (wheat, barley, and oats free) diet also. While his progress was slow, we began to see the child we knew earlier in the year reemerge. He had once again begun laughing and responding to family members.

Dietary intervention has made tremendous strides in its application to autism. Much has been done to show a link between food allergies/ intolerances and autism. While some people feel dietary intervention is a magic cure for autism, you must keep things in perspective. If your child has food allergies or intolerances, this will affect your child in some way. The theory is that in some children, like our son Nathan, their bodies process food improperly and produce toxins, even opiates that affect their brains and development. If this is allowed to continue, it can produce autistic behaviors.

You must remember that if your child is affected by food, he may have other sensitivities or deficits that are contributing to his autism. Each of these areas needs to be addressed. Nathan has quite a few tactile sensitivities, which we continue to address with his occupational therapist. He also displays obsessive tendencies, which are addressed in behavior therapy. If his food allergies are at the root of his other problems, then as the offending substance leaves his body, these things should improve. If the food is not the cause of these behaviors, then we have not wasted six months waiting for his diet to work because we have continued his therapies and our parent plan. It is common for autism diets to address gluten and casein intolerances, but soy and eggs may also be contributing factors.

A recommendation of dietary intervention is probably one of the last things a therapist or team wants to suggest to a family and does not usually make the decision light heartedly. A child with autism often has a restricted diet due to tactile, taste, or smell sensitivities. I worried that removing foods from Nathan's diet would cause my already small child to lose weight. In fact, the opposite happened. Nathan's body was able to process his food properly and gain weight.

As a parent, I would like to offer some suggestions to help encourage your child to eat. A nutritionist may not agree with all I say, but realistically, you need to feed your child, so I will just tell you what works for me. Keep in mind I do believe in good nutrition, as well as limiting snacks and processed foods. My little ones love any type of beans, especially garbanzo beans, as well as fresh spinach. When you have a child on a casein-free (dairy-free) and gluten-free (wheat-free) diet, you must remove any trace of the offending foods. This means reading labels and knowing the different forms of any names they go by. Also, just because something is wheat-free does not mean it is free of gluten. You can get this information from a nutritionist or from literature specifically about this type of diet. You may find useful information in books about Celiac's disease. People with this type of disease are unable to eat gluten. Keep in mind that they can eat dairy products, so if you use gluten-free recipes from these resources, make substitutions if necessary.

A nutritionist or pediatrician may tell you your child will eat if he gets hungry enough. As a parent, I do not find this to be true for every child. A child with sensitivities is not necessarily being stubborn and refusing to eat because of choice. I have had a child dry heave and become lethargic due to not eating, even though there was an abundance of food available. This child had to regain her interest in food and is now a healthy eater. I admit there is a fine line between refusal and ability, and the job to distinguish between the two lies on your shoulders. Trust yourself and allow for mistakes when training or retraining your child to eat.

When your child is refusing food due to food sensitivities or refusals, you may find it beneficial to keep things simple. Offer one type of food at a time. Offer variety upon completion of the first item or at the next meal. A child with autism may find order and predictability in foods left in their original form. Instead of giving your child apple slices, try giving him the whole apple. If he is young, peel the apple to discourage choking, and always supervise. This type of eating problem may be caused by the perception that the food is broken. Your child may thrive on the stimulation of his toast being cut into small pieces, while another child may feel their food has been broken or damaged. Mixing foods may be causing sensory overload. A child may not like blueberry waffles but may love plain ones. Changing or altering a food, especially a favorite one, can trigger a refusal, not only to the new food but to the food in its original form.

When Nicole was about six years old, I used milk chocolate chips in chocolate chip cookies instead of semisweet, and she did not like it. To her, it was a significant change, and it changed her perception of the cookie. Years later, she still says she does not like chocolate chip cookies despite numerous attempts at tasting them. I have observed this same behavior with other changes in her food.

Learning what your child likes and how he eats has most likely taken a toll on your family. Adding the restrictions of a special diet may seem overwhelming. But I promise you, the benefits of finding and treating food intolerance outweighs the compromises your family will make. While there are many recipes available, I do recommend the prepared mixes you find in the health food stores. These mixes have been tried and tested. If time allows you to experiment, and wasting ingredients on a failed attempt does not concern you, take the opportunity to try recipes. As you buy a mix, look at it to see what ingredients you will need to add to it. Many will list appropriate substitutes. Don't forget to check your labels. Many of these mixes will tell you that the product freezes well. The muffins and cookies we have made have done great frozen in freezer bags. This makes for easy removal of one at a time. Defrosting in the microwave for a few seconds will bring them back to tempting form. It is also recommended that any baked goods that are gluten-free be placed in the microwave before eating to improve the taste. Due to a variety of reasons we are seeing a surge in gluten free literature in mainstream media. There is an increase in the number and variety of products in our stores that are intended for those following a gluten free or gluten and casein free diet.

If you find yourself eating out or on the go, most food establishments have an ingredient list available to you. If you ask if something is gluten-free or casein-free, the server will likely not know, but he may be able to provide an ingredient list for you. Always be aware of possible cross contamination if the item is not sold as "gluten free".

As your child is on this diet, you will likely find that he will actually lose his craving for many foods he is not allowed to have. When altering your child's diet, make sure he is not using drinks to curb his hunger. One way to discourage filling up with drinks is to not offer the drink immediately at the beginning of a meal or right before mealtime. Limiting liquids is not a good idea, but you can adjust when you give the drink. If you are unsure of the amount of liquid your child should be drinking, please consult your pediatrician or a nutritionist and learn the signs of dehydration.

Mrs. Luck: Your particular dietary interventions may involve elimination of artificial coloring or flavoring, substances which may adversely affect a child's behavior. The FDA puts warning labels on these additives for a reason. For example, "This product contains FD&C Yellow No. 5 (tartrazine) which may cause allergic-type reactions (including bronchial asthma) in certain susceptible persons."[20]

Food labels will advise you if artificial colorings are added. In our home, one particular item we avoided was Red No.40 because it triggered such unwanted behavior in such a short time after ingestion. Besides being an ingredient in so many candies and snack foods, it is actually in many children's vitamins and medicines. It seems ironic that items meant to promote our child's health and well-being can have such a negative impact.

Shelli: I love essential oils. I wish that I had them from the start of my family, wait—even before I had my own family to look after. My family is amazing, and they deserve the best. I believe that the use of oils to take care of your family's health and over all wellness is the best investment you will ever make.

Before we knew anything about autism, or that we would have two children with autism, my son Joshuah had a lot of trips to the doctor. He was getting sick often, and ear infections were prominent. Each time that the doctor would send in a script for an antibiotic, I would grit my teeth. I knew it would make the infection go away and stop that pain. I also knew it would take about a month before Joshuah would be back to his normal-functioning level. I was keenly aware that the treatment would be followed by awful yeast infections. Then, I would have to get a topical antibiotic to clear that up. So many times I went to the doctor knowing in my gut that something was wrong with my son and the doctors would tell me that he was just having a bad day. We would leave, and a couple of days later, we would be back with Joshuah running 103– 104 degree temps. Sometimes, Joshuah's eardrums would not be red enough for them to give him anything just yet. Boy, I would really get frustrated. I knew my son so well; I knew when something was not right. Soon, I got frustrated enough that I took matters into my own hands. I researched homeopathic healing. I was ready to try anything that was better than what we were receiving through our pharmacy. But the cost and the time it took me to make herb-based solutions hindered me from using them. I was scared I would not be doing it right (stupid), and it was not a cost effective solution for me. So I tried to start an herb garden, which I am still attempting to do. I don't have a green thumb; I seem to kill the plants. I met a mom who started talking with me about essential oils.

She explained to me that instead of me growing oregano, thyme, rosemary, coriander, and so on, I could get the oils from those plants. I could put the oils in the food I was cooking. I could put lavender right on the bug bites that itched or my child's painful sunburns with no fear of harmful chemicals. So I began to use them. They work. For headaches, I don't reach for a bottle of Tylenol or Advil. I reach for a bottle of peppermint. It works. I was surprised at the changes I was seeing in my health and the health of my family. I'll ask someone in passing how they are doing, and if they say, "Oh, I have a headache or a cough" or "I have a sore throat," I will say, "Hey, I have an oil for that. Let me go get it." These are people that have been taking over the counter medications for the past week and their cold, cough, headache, or sore throat has not let up. I give them oils. Every time, I get hugs and praise.

When Joshuah seems to be getting an earache, I put some lavender oil and tea tree oil on a Q-tip and let it run down into his ear. It does such a great job that if his ear starts hurting again later, Joshuah will bring me my bag of oils for me to help him again. Izzy takes the oils too. Izzy has really sensitive skin, so at night, I put a little lavender oil in her bath to help clear up those rashes she gets from irritants in her environment. We also use a lot of clove oil on her. As she struggles with the anxiety that comes along with the challenges of autism, she will bite and chew on her lips until they bleed. If I put a touch of clove oil on her lips, the blister will clear up quickly.

Essential oils are antimicrobial, antibacterial, and antifungal, so you can use them to clean your home and purify the air. I use lemon with some distilled water to clean my kitchen and bathroom. If I add a touch of vinegar to that combo, I get a great natural window cleaner. If I need furniture polish I can take some olive oil and mix it with wild orange or lemon, and it polishes and sanitizes wood furniture great. Using natural ingredients means you can throw out all those harmful chemicals that are harming our families and pets. As your family is breathing in the aroma of the oils, they are also getting the therapeutic benefits as well.

Doctors' offices are starting to diffuse oils into the air in their offices to cut down on bacteria being passed around. Dentist offices diffuse lavender to calm the nerves of incoming patients getting ready for various procedures.

I truly believe that taking time to learn about essential oils is one of the best investments you can make. Trying them is a priceless investment in your family's health.

Dr. B: There are some common diets, and some really weird diets and dietary supplements are being promoted out there. My best advice is to read the dietary research of the diet you are considering and discuss your questions and concerns with your doctor. If you are going to try a diet, do it right and do it wholeheartedly. Otherwise, your child may not get the benefit of the diet. Be patient with the diet you choose. Most doctors say it takes months to see significant results. Only eliminate one food at a time, or you won't be able to determine which food was really the offending factor. I have seen hopeful parents jump from diet to diet without giving any of them time to really make an effect. At one point in our school, we had a child who could only eat nuts due to allergies and dietary restrictions. At the same time, we had another child deathly allergic to being around nuts. To keep all of the children safe and well-nourished, we all had to work together to find solutions.

Many children on the spectrum have comorbidities (other medical issues) and are often taking either supplements or pharmaceuticals for the "other" issues they present. The high prevalence of ADD or ADHD leads to many children being on medications to control the behaviors and help the child focus. Others may be on pharmaceuticals for seizure disorders, gastrointestinal issues, or sleep disorders. There are a wide variety of chemicals and biological treatments being used by parents in a search for a cure.

Doctors may discuss with you a variety of drugs or supplements to reduce self-injurious behavior, anxiety, or other troublesome symptoms of autism. Together, with your doctor, you will plan a program to meet your child's needs.

To help you sort through the various types of behavioral, learning, or biomedical treatments for autism look for large, controlled studies to validate claims made by proponents of any system, product, or medicine.

SECTION V

Schools

Autists are the ultimate square pegs, and the problem with pounding a square peg into a round hole is not that the hammering is hard work. It's that you're destroying the peg.

—Phil Collins

Choosing a School

Dr. B: Caring parents want their children to have the best education possible no matter what the child's functional abilities are. The quality of any school depends on many variables. The factors that are important to you in your situation may differ from the variables that are important to the next family. You may be lucky enough to live in a progressive school district that provides a quality education for all children. Public schools have the advantage of being free to attend and often provide transportation for children with special needs. A private school you might be considering, while costly, may have scholarships available. There are many things to consider if you are deciding between public school and private school. One positive thing about public schools is that they are held to state and federal standards. They must hire teachers with a set standard of certification qualifications. Private schools are not held to that standard. Private schools may or may not have state credentials. If that is important to you, determine the facts. If they seem to skirt around the answer or if you have any doubt, check with the state department of education. I know of a private school that would give parents misleading answers about their certification. After years of attending the school, when some students were transitioning back to public school, parents discovered their credits would not transfer. Of course, by that time, the former director who had made those promises was no longer associated with the school.

Whatever setting you are considering, take a tour of the school. This will be a great time for you to ask questions of the principal or admission director. It is also a good time to just look around at how the school operates.

Shelli: I visited one school that assured me they were equipped to handle Joshuah. On the tour, I was shown all of the "other" classrooms first. The principal was proud of these rooms. It showed in her voice. The classrooms looked and smelled clean and had beautifully colored walls. They were well lit. I could see why this principal was pleased with these rooms. We came to the last portion of the tour, and we walked to the back end of the school, down a long hallway. Two classrooms sat side by side. They were dark and not well kept. Lights were off, they had old furniture in them, and the kids were just lying around. No teaching was evident. I did not see any calendars or picture schedules posted. It looked like storage was really low because most of the walls were covered with Tupperware containers, with things just thrown on the tops of them. Let me add that I had called ahead of time to schedule an appointment for the tour, and this was the time the principal picked as the best time to visit. This was not a surprise visit. When my husband and I got to the car, my husband said to me, "Does Joshuah have to go here?" I said, "No, and he won't."

Dr. B: Ask about the teacher certifications. Private schools may have more control over class size and over the curriculum that is taught. Because the teachers are not mandated to have a state teaching certificate, they may actually come from a varied, enriched background. If you determine that a private school best meets your needs and the cost is not a factor, you might look at a day school or possibly a boarding school.

Boarding schools provide an intense twenty-four-hour, live-in therapy environment. That time commitment can help a child improve quickly. The school will have the consistent structure that some children require. Even a short placement could mean great improvements in a child's functioning. Boarding school can provide a respite for the parents while the child lives at the school. You will want to carefully investigate the school to be sure it is a good fit for your child.

Still another option is homeschooling. I have been surprised at how many families of ASD children strongly consider this option. True, it is difficult to find the ideal school options. Many parents feel protective and are afraid of the social situation their children will encounter in school. Homeschooling is difficult if you do it well, even with typical children. People who claim "homeschooling" but, in actuality, do not spend much time teaching are doing a great disservice to their children. Special needs compound the difficulty and the commitment.

Shelli: Some people reading this would gasp at the thought of homeschooling children who are diagnosed with autism. My children are lucky enough to go to a great school now. I have to say, however, that like many of you, I am a mother hen with my little chicks. I want them with me all the time. I want to protect them from sunup to sundown. I have very strong values I long to impart to my children. I love the idea of homeschooling. I think it is a beautiful concept. However, we already work with our children 24-7 without a break, going from therapy to therapy. I loved the thought of homeschooling even before I learned my children would have autism challenges. I want them to feel normal or typical. I want someone to actually teach them. I want my children to love learning. I want them to seek out learning for themselves. I want to cultivate creative learning styles. I do not want my child to be put in a classroom only to be contained so as not to disrupt the "typical" kids from their learning because they were the "bigger deal." However, parents need to sleep at some time, right? I know I do. My children tag team at night. I finally get one to sleep, and the other will start screaming. I can get that one calmed down and the first would wake up again and on and on until light starts cracking through the window, and I give up. The commitment it takes to homeschool any child is time-consuming, but one (or two in my case) on the spectrum could have detrimental effects on my own mental and physical health.

Dr. B: Whether you decide on public or private school, you will want to determine what therapies are provided at the school. Do they use the ABA therapy methods? What ancillary therapies are offered? You may need to know what the situation is for care of children before and after school hours. Are all these services included in the basic tuition, or are they add on charges? Is transportation included?

Talk to the director or principal about the basis of instruction happening in the school. Does the teaching focus on academics? Are children grouped by intelligence? Is the instruction language based or cognition based? Do they use multisensory teaching methods? Most special needs children learn best in multisensory teaching settings.

Ask what choices the child has in the school. Are there electives? What electives might apply to your child? Look at the teacher-to-student ratio in the classrooms and the daily schedule. Do the children stay in a homeroom with an assigned teacher all day, or do they move through the halls to a different classroom each hour? Could your child handle that kind of transitioning? Hall transfers are difficult for children who do not like change or are bothered by noise or chaos. Transferring classes means a different teacher for each class period, different faces, and perhaps more importantly, different voices. Will the school allow your child a modification to make the hallway time less traumatic? Would they allow him to change classes just a few minutes before or after the rest of the crowd?

The more intense your child's needs, the more attention he will need. Is every child in the school working toward his own individual goals? Or it is large class instruction with the same expectations for all? What is being done to promote thinking strategies? Do you see "hands-on activities" happening with every subject? Look to see how much support staff is being used and in what manner. Paras can be a great extension of the teacher.

What is the general atmosphere of the school? Does it seem clinical, or is it more homelike? The lunch area is sometimes a good place to get a feel of the school atmosphere. Do the children seem happy and engaged? Does the staff seem happy and appear to be enjoying the children?

Whether or not your child is a behavior concern, you will want to know how the school deals with disruptive or major behavioral issues. Another child having a temper tantrum can put your child in danger if the school does not have a good solid plan to keep everyone safe in this situation. Is the playground time well supervised? Does the school have fingerprint background checks on every employee? As you tour the school, be visually scanning for safety issues. Are doors alarmed to monitor incoming visitors and to alert the staff should a child decide to leave? If something doesn't seem quite right, ask questions. Look beyond the beautiful decorations or fancy equipment. Don't assume anything.

Shelli: My point is to be proactive. Do your homework. Compare notes and experiences with other parents in your area. You know what will work for your child. You are your child's best advocate. You are his voice. The impression I got from that school we toured and that principal was they didn't see any potential in these children, so why put forth an effort? They all deserve better than a dark room at the back of the building.

Programming

Dr. B: Once you have decided what school your child will attend, you will begin working with your school to design your child's program. The foundation of his program will be a legally binding document known as the IEP (Individualized Educational Program). The IEP is developed based on testing and observations. It will be created by a team, and you should be an important member of that team. The IEP needs to document what will be taught and in what method. It will lay out behavioral consequences, if necessary. It should identify what your child needs academically, socially, and to develop his life skills. All his ancillary therapies will be included in this master plan, as well as transportation. It will document how and when the progress will be recorded.

The team will get back together at least annually but can meet to discuss the plan before that time is up if you ask for a meeting. The evaluations and testing that form the groundwork for the plan must be updated every three years. If you think your child's evaluation isn't accurate, you have a right to request an independent evaluation, at district expense. That second opinion will be done by a professional from outside the school district. You will be notified in writing in advance of the annual and tri-annual meetings. If you cannot attend at the assigned time, ask to have the meeting rescheduled. Most schools will make an effort to work within your time constraints. You will be given copies of all documents and written copies of your rights as a parent.

Mrs. Luck: You have a right to bring an attorney or an "advocate" to the meeting. Be cautioned that in my experience, those people tend to come with a predetermined adversarial mind-set and can set a hostile tone for the meeting. If you bring a knowledgeable attorney or advocate whose intention is to work together to create an excellent program for your child, that is helpful. Some attorneys or advocates seem so intent on showing that they can bully the school that your child actually becomes a pawn in their power play.

I have heard horror stories about schools being resistive to offering a good, reasonable child-centered plan. A mom recently told me she visited the special education office in a small town seeking services for her preschool aged son who has autism. The special education director told her the only thing wrong with her son was that she stays home with him instead of going to work. The director told her if she would just put him in day care, he would "learn to behave." The only services he offered her was to bus her little guy to a town thirty miles away where he would be in a school-aged special education program for children with a mixture of diagnoses. She felt totally bullied and insulted by the man. Because the school district was so unwilling to even explore appropriate options, I gave her the phone number of a good special education lawyer and urged her to call for a consultation.

Elizabeth: "They" say never cry in an IEP meeting. Keep your emotions in check. I ask what alternate universe "they" live in. You will likely meet in a conference room with those who serve your child. You are meeting with a team that you have built to bring about success to your child, and you talk about that success. Then you talk about what has not been successful. You may have to tell those that you have built a relationship with that the service they are providing is falling short. You are flooded with information about your child's accomplishments and failures. You want it all but know that isn't possible. So you prepare by bringing your own support. A family member, a friend, a therapist, or your child's support coordinator can offer you strength at this time. The boys' current coordinator takes incredible notes and has great insight because she sees my children as individuals across different environments. Then, if tears come, don't be afraid to clarify the reason for those tears. If they come from pride, tell them you are so proud of your child. If you are sad, tell them you fear missed opportunities. Try not to be too free with your tears. Don't let them distract from writing the best plan for your child. Don't be embarrassed if they come. And wear waterproof mascara just in case.

Mrs. Luck: I have seen teachers, therapists, and principals work hard to put together a good plan for a child. The parent comes to the meeting with a chip on her shoulders, ready to do battle and demanding services that may not even be appropriate. She may bring an attorney and a list of demands that she heard that another family received from the school for *their* child. I've heard of parents who read a story about a child who showed improvement after he had a session of swimming with the dolphins, and they come to the IEP demanding that the school pay for dolphin therapy for their child.

Not every child needs the same modifications, and sometimes, a parent's demands can even be detrimental to the child's development. A common example is the hiring of a personal attendant to be with the child throughout the day. There are times that this is necessary for the safety of the child and others. However, a parent who comes to a meeting insisting that the school provide a full day personal attendant for a well-behaved honor student with Asperger's may not be considering the negative social affects. Just because someone else had a certain modification does not mean you should demand it also. Bring well thought out ideas rather than random demands.

Mrs. Nic: I have seen the best results for a good child-centered IEP when both sides work together. The parents can facilitate this by coming to the meeting with the assumption that both you and the school have the child's best interest in mind. The parent's input should be highly valued and used to help create the plan. The mom and dad know the child's needs, his triggers, and what he responds to as a reinforcer. This is a good time for parents to advocate for your child. In most cases that I have seen, it did not have to be done in an adversarial manner. The sad truth is that schools are pinched for funding. They are trying to stretch the dollar to provide for many students. In some cases, this is an overriding factor but not in every case. If no agreement can be reached, the law provides an avenue for the parent to follow as an appeal process.

If you are having a disagreement between parents and the school over any type of issue, I strongly urge both sides not to discuss it in front of the child. Like a child who finds himself in the middle of a divorce, the student will have a difficult time splitting his loyalties and performing at optimum. The unresolved issue is between the adults. The child has no means to resolve the conflict, so be careful not to put the burden on him by discussing it within earshot of him, even if you think he is not capable of understanding the conversation.

Dr. B: One of the biggest decisions in many cases is whether to place the child in a special education classroom, a typical classroom, or a combination of both. There are different terms involved in incorporating students with special needs in to the classroom of typically developing students. *Mainstreaming* is the term used to describe when students whose primary placement is in a special education class attend regular education classrooms for some part of the day. Inclusion describes the situation when students with disabilities have their primary placement in regular education classes with age matched peers. In both mainstreaming and inclusion the student will likely have some mandated modifications to promote their success.

The mandated modifications are determined individually for each child. The modifications may range from preferred seating (to minimize distractions) to visual supports (schedule, handouts, etc.)

Mrs. Nic: I sometimes see parents who are so determined to have their child in full inclusion that they are blind to the individual needs of the child. It is great for some children and a poor option for others. The typical classroom may have close to thirty students with one teacher. If she is lucky, she will have one classroom aide. She probably has little or no specialized training in working with students with special needs. Consider the fact that she would have gotten her degree in special education and be teaching in a special education class if that were where her heart lies.

SECTION VI

Resources

Gather in your resources, rally all your faculties, marshal all your energies, focus all your capacities upon mastery of at least one field of endeavor.

—John Haggai

Know Your Rights

Dr. B: By state and federal law, you have rights that are guaranteed under several different laws. There are rights assured by laws that cover special education. Your child has other rights that are covered by laws discriminating against him in the broader realm. Federal civil rights laws ensure equal opportunity for people with disabilities.

There are certain things a public school must do for special education placement of any kind. These are called Parental Procedural Safeguards. The school district will provide you with the complete document. Consult your school district or an attorney for clarification. We are not attorneys and are not giving legal advice; we are just going to highlight some of the rights you have as a parent as we interpret them.

Parents have the right to copies of their child's educational records. When an IEP meeting is held, you have the right to participate in that meeting and have your voice heard. You may bring any person who has knowledge about your child to an IEP meeting including advocates and attorneys. This might be your caseworker.

If the school district is considering a change in placement, you have a right to be notified in advance of the meeting. You may request that your child be assessed for special education services without delay. If you disagree with the testing, you have a right to ask for a second opinion. If an IEP is in place, parents have a right to request a new IEP meeting to consider changes. Parents have the right to consent, refuse to consent, or revoke consent for special education for their child. Parents who disagree with parts or all of the IEP may file due process complaints.

The federal government has established the ADA (Americans with Disabilities Act) to protect the rights of disabled persons. There are various sections to the act, giving different protections.

Title I deals with employment practices for certain companies. It prohibits discrimination in recruiting, hiring, promoting, training, pay, social activities, and other details of employment. It limits the questions that can be asked about an applicant's disability before a job offer is made. The law requires that certain employers make reasonable accommodation to the known physical or mental limitations of otherwise qualified individuals with disabilities.

The second section, Title II, requires that state and local governments give people with disabilities an equal opportunity to benefit from all of their programs, services, and activities (e.g. public education, employment, transportation, recreation, health care, social services, courts, voting, and town meetings).

Title III requires certain businesses open to the public to ensure that individuals with a disability have equal access to all that the businesses have to offer. This covers a wide range of businesses.

Title IV mandated a nationwide system of telecommunications relay services to make the telephone network accessible to people who are deaf or hard of hearing or who have speech impairments.

There are attorneys who specialize in assisting people with disabilities. Within that group, you can find lawyers who focus on special education law and others who specialize in ADA cases.

Respite Care

Dr. B: Having a family member with any type of special needs, including autism, can be a challenge. Caregivers have little time to themselves, and sometimes, it seems that the demands never end, even during the night. They can get overstressed as they deal with their family's needs, juggle school, therapy, and medical appointments. To manage financially, they may even be working outside the home. Add in special social activities for the children, fundraisers, and meetings. The rest of the family has needs to be addressed also.

Parents sacrifice their own health and well-being to meet the needs of their children in such demanding situations. Respite care is just having someone take over your caregiver duties for a time. A respite caregiver is a person who takes over, allowing you to take a break. The break could be a few minutes, or hours, or it could be a week or more. It may be time to allow you to go to the grocery store, attend a wedding, or perhaps a funeral.

Respite services can make a significant positive difference in the lives of families. It allows the caregiver to take a much needed break. Respite has been shown to have a positive impact on relationships within a family. Many parents never take that break. They may feel guilty leaving the house while someone else cares for the child. They may feel the only way they can protect their child is to be with them constantly. They wonder what people will think if they are seen out having a good time or going to a happy event such as a wedding or a birthday party while their child is at home. They worry about being judged by others, yet they judge themselves far more harshly. Perhaps the guilt stems from already feeling guilty about their situation for one reason or another. Everyone deserves a break. To have some time to yourself will allow you to return refreshed.

Who can you call upon for that needed break? Options vary depending upon your needs and the needs of your child. It's often possible to call on friends, family, or a competent adult baby sitter in order to have a short time away from the house. Caregivers may be available through your place of worship or through local agencies such as your state's Developmental Disabilities Council or other agencies or programs.

Respite care is often, but not always, given in your own home. It may be services at a day care center, agency, or camp, for example. With the high divorce rate among couples with a child on the spectrum, your respite care may be simply time that the child goes to stay with the noncustodial parent. Let the child's other parent know they must step up and do their part in the parenting of this special needs child.

Mrs. Luck: I know a single mom who has two daughters. Eight-year-old Emily is quite severely ASD.

The girl is nonverbal, demanding, and easily becomes violent. Nine-year-old Mari goes to sleepovers at her friends' houses but is not comfortable having her friends stay over at her house. The mom's attention is very often consumed with tending to Emily's needs. However, every year on Mari's birthday weekend, the mom arranges respite care for Emily at a caregiver's home. Emily stays the whole weekend with the caregiver, and Mari gets her mom's full attention for the weekend. On one night of the birthday weekend, Mari hosts a sleepover for several of her friends. Mari says it is the best birthday gift she ever gets.

Mrs. Nic: You may have the advantage of a relative you know well and trust with your child. If you need to use an agency or a service, be sure the person has passed a background check, knows CPR and basic first aid, and is knowledgeable about autism. Do your research, interview extensively. Let the caregiver spend time with you and your child before the respite date so that they get to know each other and feel comfortable. Have a copy of your information packet available and make sure the caregiver understands the house rules and discipline processes. Diet, allergy, and medication information is important. Discuss your child's triggers and what items you use to reinforce good behaviors. Give them a schedule and make sure they know how important that schedule is to your child.

Shelli: My family and my in-laws are the people I call on for respite care when I need it. If one of them can't come, another one will. I feel so good leaving my children in their hands, even if it is just for me to go to another room for a couple of hours of desperately needed sleep. My children sense the trust and love I feel for the family members and they are totally comfortable with the respite.

Camps

Dr. B: Another type of respite you may consider as your child gets a little older is camp. The challenge is to find the right camp for your child. Depending on where you live, there may be very few choices, or you may have many choices and, therefore, decisions to make. There are sleepaway camps, day camps, special-interest camps, and camps that focus mainly on social skill development. Some might be right in your own neighborhood, but others that meet your needs might be a long drive from home. Some camps are highly structured while others give the campers ample free time. Social development, personal growth, and independence are goals of many of the camps for special needs children.

You will need to do your homework to find camps that meet your child's needs. Word of mouth from other parents is a great way to find out about camps. Another good tool is the internet.

One decision you will face is whether you want an inclusive camp or a special services camp. There are camps such as Camp Barnabas in Southwest Missouri that assign camper week by the child's diagnosis. This allows them to be correctly staffed and to plan activities matched to the particular diagnosis. At Camp Barnabas, certain weeks are set aside for ASD campers. Other camps, such as Camp Encourage just outside of Kansas City, are specifically designed to meet the needs of children on the spectrum.

Whether to choose a day camp or a sleepaway camp is a big decision. You are the best judge of your child's ability to handle the overnight situation. Remember, the counselors and volunteers at the specialty sleepaway camps are specially trained to help the camper adjust to the situation. Cabins are usually divided by age group and gender.

After you investigate the camp situation, you will fill out an application. The application process will entail giving extensive medical and educational information to the camp staff. At most camps, the camp counselor assigned to your child will then make a personal call to your camper to meet him over the phone. Even if your child is nonverbal, the counselor will introduce himself in this phone meeting. As the child listens, the counselor will tell the camper what to expect at camp and will outline the activities the child can take part in. This helps the camper transition to the camp. One counselor told of her call to Alex, a new camper. He did not say a word as she talked about the camp. His mom later reported that when the call ended, Alex bounced off walls whooping and hollering that he was so excited now about camp. He talked compulsively for the next month about the fact that he was going to camp and was going to go swimming.

Mrs. Nic: Camp can be a profound experience for a child. To help a camper on the spectrum prepare for camp, I have seen parents provide a countdown calendar to mark off the days until it is time to go. Children will enjoy having a brochure or a web page showing the camp. They can look at the activities and the camp surroundings. If you provide your child with a picture of the counselor assigned to him, that can be helpful. Structured activities such as making a printed list of items to pack for camp are reassuring for the camper. It lets him feel prepared and assured that he has everything he needs to pack when it is time to check in at camp. Some campers feel more comfortable if they go to camp together with a friend.

Elizabeth: There are some glorious camps in our area. Although my friends swear by them, I haven't been brave enough to even consider sending Nathan. I might consider sending Chase, who is just now getting old enough to go. I have even thought of sending them together to have Chase keep an eye on Nathan and provide a feeling of security for Nathan. When the thoughts creep in, I do remember my brother. He went to MDA camp each year. It was an incredible time for him. Camp was a time of joy and independence. I remember the last year my brother went. He cried because it was his last year. He was too old to return. And truly it was his last year. He passed away that fall. But the memories of him coming home and telling us about his experience remains strong. Listening to stories about campfires and warm fuzzies is what I think about when I think about camp. I want that for my sons.

Dr. B: A great feature of most specialty camps is the "peer models." Typical teenagers attend the camp with the special needs campers and serve as role models. They blend in with the campers, take part in all activities, and lead the way.

Elise, a camp counselor, shared with me her experience with campers on the spectrum paired with peer models:

Kevin was a sixteen-year-old camper diagnosed with autism. He was a very quiet boy and the only time I'd hear him speak was when he was pacing in the back of the cabin singing with his MP3 player. He didn't interact much with the other kids but always participated in the activities as requested. One morning, our cabin decided to go fishing in a pond located at the campsite. Each camper was paired with a peer model. I gave each camper/peer model a fishing pole and bait and then just monitored for any difficulties. We paired Kevin with Tony, a fifteen-year-old peer model. Shortly after they started fishing, I noticed Tony grab the pole from Kevin to work with the line, and from a distance, it appeared that he hooked something. He then handed the pole back to Kevin and said, "Never mind. It swam away."

I really didn't think anything of it until a few seconds later when Tony began encouraging Kevin to reel the line in. Kevin started jumping with joy when he realized a fish was on that line. Suddenly, Kevin, who was always quiet, became overjoyed and went around yelling, "I caught a fish!"

To this day, Kevin thinks he is the one who caught that fish, which is exactly what Tony wanted him to feel. All the counselors and fellow peer models started crying out of joy. The minute Kevin's mom returned to camp, he let her know about the fish he caught. She began to cry and hug us while telling us that Kevin had never caught a fish before. This story and these two boys will always have a special place in my heart. Kevin got to feel success while fishing. Tony got to have an opportunity to help a peer with special needs. This story really embodies what the camp experience can be like for individuals on ASD.

Another incident at camp touched my life. I was the counselor for the teenage boys. It was Ethan's second year of camp. One afternoon, he had an unexpected seizure in the pool when playing pool basketball with peer model Nate. By the time we all realized what was going on, Nate had already flipped Ethan over so his face wasn't down in the water and got the attention of the lifeguard. I remember my heart sinking when I saw Ethan. By this point, I knew him well enough to know his seizures mortified him. I was afraid he was going to shut down during the remainder of camp and want to go home. In addition to that, peer model Nate at the age of fourteen had just successfully responded to his new best friend having a seizure.

When Ethan came around, he was surprisingly calm about his seizure. All the campers, especially those on the spectrum, came to Ethan with kind words and began sharing their own stories. I sat back and listened to these kids discuss their seizure experiences. I had never seen a group of teenagers on the spectrum get together and talk like that with each other. The majority of them could relate to Ethan, and I saw in that moment how camp helped them. There was something in each and every one of them that they understood about each other. I could never do for Ethan what those kids did for him that day. That is where my love for camps and peer groups really stemmed from.

Funding

Dr. B: The Autism Society cites estimates of $3.2 million for the lifetime costs of caring for a person with autism. Parents of children with ASD face years of immense costs for treatments and services. For many families, it doesn't take long to exhaust their finances. Sometimes, help is available to some families through their medical insurance. With just over 60 percent of the states now mandating that insurance coverage be extended to cover autism, this is a relief to some households. Not surprisingly, there are significant loopholes to the mandate. You may want to investigate the possibility of obtaining double coverage. Some of our families are covered by the medical insurance through their employer, and they purchase child-only policies through another source. Whether that additional policy is with a private insurance company or with Medicaid, the cost of the premiums involved may well be offset by the added benefits of the secondary insurance. Be resourceful and investigate all options.

Check to see if your child qualifies for SSI. Supplemental Security Income (SSI) benefits are given to some children with disabilities. Investigate whether your child can take advantage of that program. Your school will often help you with this by writing letters of support.

Some parents are talented as to using the internet and their networking connections to locate charitable foundations with available grants to help families offset the costs of treatments. In most states, there is some public funding available. Finding it is not usually fast and the application processes are often time consuming, so be diligent and patient. Your caseworker may be able to help. Don't be shy about bringing resources to her that you would like her to help you access. Many caseworkers will pursue avenues that they know about, but they may not be familiar with a wide variety of funding sources.

Some employers will give a charitable donation to help an employee's child cover the medical or educational expenses. They may have a certain amount of money earmarked annually for charitable donations and may be happy to donate to your child's cause. I have seen some employers give a one-time donation, and others help a family on a monthly basis.

Don't be afraid to reach out and ask for financial support. I knew a family who had monthly stipends from ten different sponsors to help cover the costs of a special school. A few of the donors were family members who each gave a small donation each month. This was supplemented by a check from her employer and another from a friend. Even her dentist sent in a check each month to help with the expense of her private school. None of the ten checks that came in monthly was huge, but they were consistent. When they were all added together, it made the difference she needed to stay enrolled in the school of her choice.

Mrs. Nic: I know several families who get some financial support from their churches. In some of the cases, the financial help was limited to a one-year commitment, but that was certainly appreciated. One family I have worked with approached the fraternities and sororities of our local university. They located one who was looking for a philanthropic direction and was happy to donate proceeds from a fundraiser. Since many of the children with ASD have other health issues, remember to search for help which may be available for the co-morbidities.

Mrs. Luck: Parents in local autism support groups do a lot of fundraisers. These events range from bake sales to very large galas which raise tens of thousands of dollars. Some of those monies are sent on to national research organizations or the national autism societies. Other times the funding is kept locally and is accessed for the needs of the families in our own area. The Autism Speaks website lists foundations that provide a variety of help to families.

Dr. B: As of this writing, thirty-two states have mandated that insurance companies extend certain medical benefits to cover autism, according to Autism Speaks. That leaves eighteen states where insurance companies are not banned from discriminating against persons on the spectrum. Considering the costs incurred by families seeking these services for their children, this is a huge issue.

I have met families who pack up the family and move to another state where they are more likely to obtain insurance coverage. I have met others who change jobs to obtain insurance that is more autism friendly.

Even in the states where coverage is mandated, the insurance companies I have dealt with do not make it easy. Dealing with an insurance company can take a tremendous amount of time and be unbelievably frustrating. I can only suggest you keep meticulous notes. Keep a written record of every conversation you have with the insurance company. By date, list who you spoke to and what they told you.

Elizabeth: My biggest push for bringing autism insurance to our state was not so it would cover therapy for autism, but that children with autism could get medical coverage. I was curious to see how the insurance played out. Most importantly though, I don't think the general public understands that it is common for a child with autism to be denied health insurance because they have autism, even though the policy does not cover autism therapy or even speech therapy. Our children are not magically protected from illness and disease just because they have an autism diagnosis. They still need adenoids removed, get earaches, and even have heart disease. That is why I fought for insurance coverage: to give families the ability to provide basic medical coverage for their children.

During one of my trips to the state capital, a representative asked me how he could justify to one of his supporters that he voted to increase that person's premiums to pay for something that didn't directly affect him. I said, "Tell him I helped pay for his knee replacement, his wife's breast cancer screening, and possibly his son's rehab."

When insurance legislation passed in this state, I was cautiously optimistic. We paid an additional cost rider to assure the coverage. The insurance representatives were poorly trained and uninformed. Half the time, they thought we had to meet a deductible. At other times, we ended up paying a daily copayment with nothing going to the deductible. In the end, it didn't matter because the bills weren't paid by insurance and we were forced to pull our sons from their intense therapy. So the bottom line is that it is still a work in progress. If you are waiting for coverage, I advise not waiting. Find a way or find the time to do it yourself. You cannot sit back and wait for it to get sorted out. Act now.

SECTION VII

Home Life

Call it a clan, call it a network, call it a tribe, call it a family. Whatever you call it, whoever you are, you need one.

—Jane Howard

Self-Care

D r. B: An ultimate goal for all children is for them to function independently in their completion of activities of daily living, such as dressing, eating, grooming, and taking care of their bathroom needs. It is well understood that many children with autism will experience significant difficulty in their development of those self-help skills. Social, behavioral, and communication deficits that define autism all factor into the difficulties these children may have in developing those skills. Adequate self-help skills are critical for maintaining physical health and social acceptance.

Toilet training children on the spectrum carries unique problems for parents and professionals. The children have a wide variety of self-help abilities. As with typical children, some will learn more quickly than others. Learning characteristics that are considered to be common to autism can be advantageous to learning independent routines. People with autism often enjoy completing familiar routines and can remember precise sequences of events. The sensory problems some children face can actually be a benefit when it comes to grooming.

They may be sensitive to the feeling of a wet or soiled diaper and be motivated to be potty trained at an early age. They may hate to have dirty hands or face and happily learn to wash themselves.

Others have a more difficult time. When designing intervention strategies, it is helpful to understand why your child with autism has difficulty completing tasks independently. When you determine which factors are relevant to your own child, you can establish a plan to help him overcome the obstacles.

Mrs. Luck: One mom told me she figured out her daughter wouldn't pee in the toilet because she hated the sound of her urine hitting the water. When Mom realized this was the barrier, she put sound reducing headphones on the little girl when the toddler was on the potty. The child was quickly toilet trained after her mom figured out what the obstacle was.

Dr. B: A child with ASD may not feel the same desire to please the parent that we see in a typical child of that age. He may not have the social motivation to be a "big boy" or take pride in that accomplishment. Social rewards may carry little meaning for him. Difficulties in comprehending language may hinder the child's ability to understand what is expected of him in potty training. Children with ASD may not understand why you want them to eliminate in the toilet as opposed to their diapers. They often have attachment to routines. They are resistant to change. These characteristics may make the transition from diapers to the toilet difficult. The child may be used to the sensation of wearing diapers and be resistant to change since they see no need for that change.

The bathroom itself may be overstimulating to them, as it normally has bright lights and sounds of running and flushing water. They may be sensitive to temperature changes they feel as they undress. The child may have difficulty interpreting his own bodily signals such as the need to eliminate.

Generally, children with autism will let you know when they are ready for toilet training. The signs we watch for are the same signs a typically developing child may show, but the signs might appear when your child is older, and the training might take longer.

The child may begin to let you know he needs to have his diaper changed. He may use words or actions to indicate this to you. Many little ones actually go to the diaper bag and bring a clean diaper to the parent. Some will even lie down and assume the position, legs high in the air. To be successful, a child should be able to follow simple directions. It is helpful if you are noticing periods of dryness, indicating the child is able to hold urine for a period of time.

Elizabeth: Please don't assume toilet training will be a hard transition. Some ASD children can be trained fairly easily at a young age. After identifying his readiness, the first step in potty training is to teach him how to communicate that he has to go to the bathroom. If your child is unable to communicate with you that he has to go to the bathroom, it will make toilet training almost impossible, and just watching for the dance is not a long-term solution. Your child may not display the typical signs of a full bladder and may not be able to read his own sensations that indicate his needs. Provide him with this tool. For those who are nonverbal, sign language is a good system. The sign for toilet is the letter *T*, made by a fist with the thumb poking up between the pointer and the second finger. Make the fist and give it a little twist. We continue to use that easy sign. Make sure his school is providing the same routine for your child.

Mrs. Nic: When they learn to give you a sign, you will need to act fast because the sign usually does not come with much warning time. I was shopping with a friend who has a toddler on the spectrum. Elli is a bright little girl. Her mom had admonished her not to pee in her pretty new big girl pants but instead be sure to tell Mommy when she needs to use the toilet. In the second store of the morning, the alarm came: "*Pee!*" Glancing around and seeing no restroom, the mom quickly asked a clerk. Ms. Clerk curtly informed us they had no public restroom. Elli's mom pleaded with the clerk to let us take the little one to a bathroom. Ms. Clerk stood firm. But her resolve was no match for Elli. This child was a rule follower. As she stood in the middle of the carpet and pulled down her pretty panties and squatted there to pee, Ms. Clerk suddenly decided they did, indeed, have a toilet this sweet child could use.

Dr. B: As we observe and analyze to determine what barriers are keeping the child from being successful, we can then start addressing toilet training in a very individualized manner.

One of your first decisions will be whether to use a potty chair or start directly with the toilet. Breaking down the task into the smallest possible tasks will help you pin point the battle ground.

For a child who resists sitting on the toilet at all, let him have success in smaller increments. Let him explore the toilet or potty chair and practice sitting on it with his clothing on. He may spend a little time sitting on the toilet with it covered. If he appears to be afraid of the hole in the seat, cover the seat with a towel, then gradually over time remove the towel. Some parents report cutting a hole in the towel and expanding that hole a little each day. Parents have reported that modeling the desired behavior can be a powerful instructional tool. Some have used a doll to create a model for the child to follow.

If your child is frightened of the flushing sound, some parents have suggested giving an advanced warning that you are about to flush. You can wait until the child is outside of the room before you flush. Later, you can work on flushing sooner. Many children love to be the one to flush the toilet. If he has the control, that sometimes helps with the fear.

Mrs. Luck: Potty training and other grooming tasks are good situations for making use of social stories. You can make up your own, or you can find some that others are sharing online. If you need a hand with this, just ask the speech pathologist who is working with your child.

Dr. B: Learning to brush his teeth can be another challenge for your child. It is crucial to master this task in order to avoid the pain and suffering caused by cavities. Clean teeth and fresh breath are also important in the quest to be socially acceptable. If your child is having a difficult time with this task, once again, you will become the detective to determine the root cause of the avoidance. Is he overly sensitive to the stimuli involved in the process? Does he struggle with the sequencing of the steps involved?

Elizabeth: If he is struggling with brushing his teeth, tooth brushing may be a sensory issue for him. Keep this in mind instead of assuming your child just isn't learning the task. Tactile sense is your child's sense of touch. These sensitivities may be anywhere on the skin, including the inside of the mouth. Your OT or your SLP can provide you with activities to decrease oral sensitivities. Those activities and therapies will include anything that exposes your child to different types of texture, pressure, vibration, movement, and temperature.

Mrs. Luck: I think the key word here is *options*. There are many choices available to you and your child to enhance the tooth brushing experience. Explore water temperatures. Some children are less sensitive to warmer water than the cold water we normally use when brushing. Toothpaste offers many choices of texture and flavors. He may accept the feel of gel type toothpaste better than the gritty type. You can explore the various flavors that your child may like such as fruit- or bubble gum–flavored toothpaste. Sometimes, they just like the fact that their toothpaste tube has a favorite cartoon character pictured on the side of the tube.

You also have an option of what type of toothbrush works best for you and your child. Some people find a soft baby brush to be better tolerated. Others prefer the type of toothbrush that you can slip on over your finger. You can buy a two-sided toothbrush that doubles your scrubbing surface to quicken the time involved. There is even a three-sided brush available commercially. As the children bring toothbrushes to school, I notice they are all proud of which character is pictured on their toothbrush, ranging from Thomas the Tank Engine to Super Heroes.

Some children *hate* an electric toothbrush. For others, it is preferred. This will depend on his sensitivities.

Mrs. Nic: A lot of parents find that cleaning the teeth with a washcloth is a good first step. You might find yourself using this method for quite a while. Toothbrushing can be a slow process to accomplish.

Elizabeth: Bath time can be a significant challenge. Remember there is a reason for your child's behavior. Resistance to baths can be of a sensory nature. Often, a child with autism will not be able to tolerate the sound of the tub being filled. If this is the case, you may choose to close the bathroom door and to not let your child be near the bathroom as you fill the tub. Water temperature may also affect your child's response to the bath. Another thing to consider is that a past experience may cause your child to avoid bath time. If the bath was too hot or too cold for a sensitive child, it may have been a traumatic experience for them. A child with autism will overgeneralize this one experience and use it as a template for every bath. If this happened, nurture your child and try to retrain him in the basics of bath taking. I am not saying it won't be a struggle, but even blowing bubbles can be a good distraction.

The reason for a behavior may not be obvious. We battled for almost a year with Nicole's baths. We tried everything: changing temperature, not being in the bathroom as the tub was being filled, using a little water, using a lot. We got to the point where if we began washing her hair the second her foot touched the water, we could usually get through the bath. But if we even hesitated a little, we opted not to wash her hair. One day, I missed that small window of opportunity, but she needed her hair washed. Completely at my wit's end, I pleaded with her to please tell me why she screams and doesn't like her bath. That is when Nicole signed "dirty water." Those words just about knocked me over. How many times had she heard me say we wash our face first while the water is clean? To her, hair is just an extension of her face. To her, I could have been dumping mud over her head. I explained the water is not dirty, showed her the difference, and told her Mommy was sorry to make her think the water was dirty. To her credit, she believed me and understood. We never had bath problems again.

Mrs. Nic: Fear of the dirty water affects ASD children in other ways also. One boy I know prefers the shower to the bath, as he has a steady flow of clean water. If the drain starts to clog slightly and water begins to pool in the bottom of the tub he gets extremely agitated and has a total meltdown.

As children become more independent with bathing, a visual chart showing all the steps they must follow can come in handy. They may have difficulty sequencing the steps of grooming without a visual support.

Dr. B: Hair care is yet another area where your detective work will help you discover what is causing the refusal. One mom realized her son's avoidance of teeth brushing and hair grooming was the result of his fear of germs. He was afraid to touch the dreaded germs with his hands. It didn't seem to bother him that the germs were in his mouth or on his hair; he just didn't want to touch them. When she allowed him to do his daily grooming using rubber gloves his compliance showed some improvement. She tells me that hair washing has always been a battle and he doesn't mind walking around with dirty hair. However, his hair must be perfectly combed, as he can't stand to have a hair out of place.

Mrs. Luck: Haircuts are another possible battle. Again, determine the sensitivities and how you will avoid the problem. A lot of parents cut the child's hair at home as opposed to the barber shop or salon, with its smells, sounds, and strangers. Some children hate the sound of scissors snipping, yet others prefer it to the buzz of a razor. Either way, ear buds playing a favorite recording can be helpful.

Dr. B: Children with ASD may be terrified of haircuts. Some older children have described it to me as feeling like a part of them is being cut off. The same problem arises with clipping of the fingernails and toenails. Parents who realize this fear have sometimes cut hair and clipped nails while the child slept. This can be a solution for children who can't sit still long enough to get a haircut or nails clipped. A very wiggly child can end up with a disastrous haircut or a bloody fingernail.

Dressing is another area where we strongly advise the proactive parenting style that we have been describing for grooming practices. Try to determine what sets your child off about the activity and address the specific problem.

Learning how to get dressed actually begins with learning how to get undressed. Undressing is a skill most ASD children seem to figure out at a fairly early age. Many of them can strip down in a split second. Your goals here are twofold: figure out why he strips and teach him to only undress in appropriate places like a bedroom or a bathroom. The desire to shed clothing may be due to sensitivity to a fabric that irritates him. He may be annoyed by the tightness of elastic or the constriction of other fasteners on the clothing. It may be a temperature preference. He just may feel more comfortable when he feels the cool air on his naked body. To understand his motivation is your key to creating a plan to handle it.

Elizabeth: A child who is hypersensitive can be distressed by certain clothing textures. He may resist certain types of clothing. Many typical children complain of tags in clothing or seams in socks. This is more than just an irritant in children with tactile issues. Without language, they are unable to express themselves to let you know of their discomfort and how extreme it may be. This often results in a power struggle when it comes to dressing.

As you work with your child to help him become more comfortable and slowly desensitized, keep in mind that he is not simply being picky or irrational. To him, it is an issue of how things feel. Try to accommodate your child with comfortable clothing. Be careful not to encourage obsessive needs, like never putting him in clothing with elastic bands or always wearing long sleeves. By being too exact with your child's clothing, you may find your child engages in increasingly ritualistic dressing and clothing requirements. Understand his needs, but keep offering less severe textures or other irritants. Also remember your child will associate his comfort with the types of clothing he wears, so try to use a variety. Otherwise, you may end up having a child who refuses to wear anything but sweats and the same two T-shirts.

You may have a child who is seeking stimuli because of hyposensitivity. Nicole would wear up to a dozen shirts at a time because of the comfort she received from the pressure. If your child does this, layering is a good idea. But it can get out of control quickly. To help avoid this, you may choose to keep only a small amount of clothing in your child's drawer. Make only the clothing you feel is appropriate available to him. Offering therapies that provide pressure during or right before dressing your child may help decrease the need for layering or pressure from clothing. Applying slight pressure to the joints or pulling lightly on joints to release pressure and using weighted blankets or toys may provide enough deep pressure stimulation to help your child through the dressing routine. This should be done with the guidance of your occupational therapist so you will know the correct amount of pressure to apply.

Nicole loved to wear as many T-shirts as she could get on. This was often close to a dozen, and the purple one had to be the last one on. It was her favorite. There was no convincing her that this was too many. With patience and only keeping an appropriate amount in her drawer, we were able to keep this behavior under control until she was able to find other sources to fill this need. It did take some planning, and she was allowed to wear up to three shirts at a time. This kept her from going through the dirty laundry looking for more. Try to compromise with your child (this is not the same as trying to reason with him) by allowing him to fill a need but also teaching him limits and appropriate behavior. This may not happen without a fight. If your child is allowed times to fill this need, it may make the times when it is not possible easier on everyone.

Mrs. Nic: Children with autism may have difficulty with buttons or zippers due to poor fine motor skills. Clothing with as few fastenings as possible may make dressing easier. Selecting items with Velcro fastenings or large buttons and zips will allow the child to develop the fine motor skills needed to develop the ability to fasten and unfasten clothes. As time progresses, you may introduce items with smaller buttons. Another important strategy for dressing children with autism is to allow plenty of time for the activity. This is evident even when the school children are just putting on a sweater or jacket for outside play.

Mrs. Luck: They may lack the sequencing skills to remember in which order to put the clothes on. One trick in teaching a task that requires sequencing is to lay the clothes out in the order you want them to be put on. Rather than giving your child his clothes in a stacked pile, lay them out in an organized line. Unfold each item so it gives a correct visual clue of the right way to wear it. I have noticed shirts with pictures or characters on the front are easier for children who are just learning to dress themselves. That gives them information as to which side of the shirt goes in the front.

Disruptive Behaviors

Elizabeth: The coping skills that your child adopts to deal with the frustrations in his life may be positive or negative. These are the behaviors your child uses to get through an overwhelming situation or just to get through the day. Negative coping skills include but are not limited to: withdrawal, self-stimulation, and aggressive or erratic behavior. Negative coping skills produce what we commonly think of as autistic characteristics. Each of these negatives has a more appropriate positive coping skill which should be encouraged.

A child who shows signs of withdrawal could be allowed downtime. Allow your child time for listening to music, wrapping up in a blanket or weighted blanket, or any calming activity. Even sitting in a dark room to clear away the stimulants is okay at times, if it is your child's choice. This allows your child to start over and in a sense clear his head. This is different than withdrawal because your child is closing off the excessive stimulation, not the entire world by pulling into his own world and not responding to anything.

Rather than being allowed to self-stimulate, engage your child in sensory activities. Self-stimulation is not exclusively a coping mechanism. Often, it is a need for sensory input. Self-stimulating activities are things like spinning, rocking, hand flapping, and making repetitive noises. Whichever the case, sensory input and stimulation will encourage proper behaviors and will lessen the need for the self-stimulation. The child who spins continually and never falls down will likely benefit from using a scooter board. Just remember as you spin your child on the board, make sure he is responding to the environment. Otherwise, you are actually encouraging your child to continually spin.

Nicole loves the story of how we taught her to get dizzy. Like many children with autism, she did not respond to her environment when spinning in circles. She didn't focus on objects as she twirled and therefore never became dizzy or fell down. While it may seem like a talent, not noticing your surroundings creates problematic behavior, missed opportunities, and inability to read cues. That is where the scooter board came in. Nicole would sit on a scooter board surrounded by people who would request eye contact and give directives for her to look at objects in her line of sight. While we gave directives, we turned her in circles. Spinning would only continue if she gave that eye contact and didn't seem to disappear into her own thoughts. Many hours were spent doing this. Finally, she got dizzy and fell off the board. Then we celebrated.

Aggressive or erratic behavior may be how your child learned to escape. You can help your child produce positive coping skills when a situation is overwhelming by first allowing for his need for predictability. Then, help your child find ways to calm himself and find another outlet for the anxiety he is feeling. The therapies your child is engaging in will encourage tolerance in time. You and your child need to find a way to communicate to each other about the level of anxiety your child feels. He may need to be physically removed from a situation before a tantrum begins. With Nicole, she got to the point where she knew when she had to leave noisy rooms, and we left while I counted until she told me to stop. Having a means of physical escape increased her tolerance level because she was in control of the situation. While leaving should not be your ultimate goal, it is sometimes necessary. You will be helping your child learn to calm himself. A small tactile activity, like silly putty, may offer just enough of the proper stimulation and distraction to carry your child through. Headphones work well for older children, especially in an atmosphere like an airport or other chaotic environment.

Dr. B: In an online blog, an anonymous Autism-Daddy defines the difference between a temper tantrum and an autism meltdown. I think he hit the nail on the head with this description.

Tantrums Age 1–5 years	Autism Meltdowns Through adulthood
"Want" directed	Overstressed / Overwhelmed
Goal/ control driven	Reactive mechanism
Audience to perform	Continues without attention
Checks engagement	Safety may be compromised
Protective mechanism	Fatigue
Resolves when goal is accomplished	Not goal dependent May require assistance to regain control

It has become a trend in young parents to mislabel the temper tantrums of their typical child as "meltdowns." Somehow this characterization seems more socially acceptable. But in fact there is a true difference between a good old fashioned temper tantrum and an autistic meltdown, and they need to be handled differently. I think that as so many parents of typical children now attempt to minimize their child's temper tantrums by mislabeling them as *meltdowns*, the word takes on a distorted meaning.

Sleep disturbances are disruptive to both the child and the parents. If your child is not sleeping, chances are you will be sleep-deprived as well. Sleep disturbances include difficulty falling asleep, difficulty staying asleep, or a poor quality of sleep. Some medical conditions which are common in ASD children interfere with good sleep, such as respiratory problems.

A very recent study on the relationship between autism and sleep disturbances was published in the Archives of

Disease in Childhood. The authors completed what is being described as the largest study to date on this topic. They concluded that children with autism go to sleep later at night than their typical peers. They also wake earlier in the morning. This is further exasperated by the fact that they wake far more frequently during the night. The authors reported that this discrepancy begins around thirty months of age and continues until age eleven, which was the parameter of the study.[21]

There are some interesting theories about why sleep disturbances are so prevalent among this population. One thought is that the successful bedtime routine requires being able to read social clues. From an early age, a typical toddler will know when you put his pajamas on him, fix him a bottle, and start to rock him that he is expected to go to sleep. He knows what it means when other family members are preparing for bed as it gets dark outside and activity inside the house starts to wind down. Children with autism may not feel the need to conform to the patterns of the rest of the family.

Mrs. Nic: Some children learn to manipulate the bedtime routine to stall the final act of going to sleep. They might require a bath and then need a parent to read them a story. Then perhaps, they suddenly need to look for a favorite stuffed animal. A request for a drink of water might be followed by the need to use the bathroom again. After all, what parent can refuse to give a child a drink of water or allow them to use the toilet?

Dr. B: Children on the spectrum could have an increased sensitivity to outside stimuli, such as touch or sound, causing them to have trouble falling asleep or awaken in the middle of the night. While most kids continue to sleep soundly despite small sounds inside or outside of the home, a child with autism might awaken.

Some researchers theorize sleep problems in ASD children are caused by anxiety. Children with autism tend to score high on anxiety scales, and that may account for sleeplessness.

There are studies that suggest children on the spectrum have difficulty with regulation of melatonin. Melatonin is a hormone that helps regulate sleep patterns. Researchers claim some children with autism don't release melatonin at the correct times of day. Melatonin levels typically rise in response to darkness (at night) and dip during the daylight hours. Instead, ASD children sometimes have high levels of melatonin during the daytime and lower levels at night. Many parents report that sleep improved after they had a discussion with their pediatrician and implemented a regimen of melatonin. As Shelli discussed in earlier chapters, she had to be persistent with her doctor, but when he followed her lead, the results were positive.

Think back to all the advice you have heard over the years of how to establish a helpful sleep pattern. Avoidance of late-day stimulants, calming activities at bedtime, and an evening routine might help. A good family sleep schedule and daily exercise are often discussed as part of the solution. A dark, cool, quiet sleep environment is normally suggested. Although those things may not be the solution to your problem, they certainly can't hurt.

Family Life

Dr. B: Having children on the spectrum totally changes the dynamics in the home. The family routines, the interrelationships among family members, and their social contacts are all affected. I have spent time talking with siblings of ASD kids. There is no doubt in my mind that being a sibling of a child on the spectrum becomes a defining factor in his life. Most of the older siblings I have met are fiercely protective of the sibling with ASD. Yet within that protective cloak, there is often a spark of resentment for the immense amount of parental time consumed in dealing with the child with autism. Although there is deep love, they describe a family that revolves around the struggles of the child on the spectrum. Michaela is the sibling of a young man on the spectrum. I am going to share her story with you here.

> I was two years old when Dennis was born. Originally, I was not a fan of sharing the spotlight, but I soon recovered after I discovered how fun it was being an older sister. When Dennis was a toddler, I thought my brother was the coolest brother ever! I could put makeup on him and

dress him in tutus, and he wouldn't say a thing! I remember girls in my kindergarten class always telling me about their fights with their siblings, and I felt like the luckiest girl in the world. Dennis would sit in a desk all day while I played teacher. He would sit with me at the tea parties. He would never fight with me or want to change the game we were playing. I was lucky. When he started speaking, I was the only one who could understand him.

Then reality started sinking in. As fun as it was having a sibling who always did what I wanted, as I entered first grade, I started to realize this wasn't normal. My grandmother was on hospice and was spending her final days at our house. We were all sitting around her crying, and my brother was found in the corner, playing with toys. I remember some extended family members commenting that my brother was weird or emotionless.

My friends all found it annoying when he bit himself out of frustration. He wouldn't let me hug him and would go hide in his room if he hurt himself. I didn't understand why he was so different.

When I realized my brother was different and that not everybody understood, I became protective almost to the point of an unhealthy protectiveness. My brother was always obsessed with football, particularly the statistics that come with football, and wanted to join the team his freshman year. I was a senior when he entered high school and was lucky enough to be friends with the quarterback. With his help, I knew everybody on the football team, and I may have done a tiny bit of threatening to ensure my brother was treated with respect. This is so natural of siblings. I have yet to meet a person who wouldn't give an arm or a leg for their sibling on the spectrum.

As I mentioned earlier, Dennis joined the football team in high school. This terrified all of us. A lot of hormonal boys in one room seemed like a recipe for teasing disaster. However, these boys on the team were so different from the horror stories you hear about on the news. With bullying being a "hot topic," it was so inspirational to see that not all kids bully. Not only was Dennis welcomed, but he was given the nickname Easy Mac because of his resemblance to the Easy Mac kid. I remember I was terrified the very first Meet the Players night. As a senior on the dance team, I had been to a lot of Meet the Players nights. Essentially, they say your name, and you stand while your parents and friends take pictures. This is an event that one-third of our small town comes to see. Let me just say that from a high school perspective, your status in life depends on how many people cheer for you. If you got a lot of cheers, you were the coolest person in the world, pretty much. I was so worried that nobody would cheer for Dennis, and he would feel sad (he probably wouldn't have noticed, but I didn't understand this at that point). When Dennis's name was called, the whole football team and crowd stood and cheered for Easy Mac. He was the only football player who got a standing ovation that night. Everybody loved him and loved using his new nickname, and that's when I knew I didn't need to worry. It is my hope that every child on the spectrum gets to experience a standing ovation.

To this day, I am still more protective than anyone I know in regards to my brother. The day he went to college, I pulled his roommate aside and described autism and ended it with, "If you hurt him I will find you." Dennis is currently a senior at Missouri State University working toward a degree in accounting. College has had its fair share of challenges, particularly because Dennis did not have a specific diagnosis. Without a current IEP, he was unable to get modifications such as longer test time. We did have the option of having him assessed by a campus counselor to get these modifications, but Dennis is unaware of his deficits, and we worried about discussing these with him so late in his life. He is living in the dorms, though, and does continue to do well. I could not be more proud of my baby brother.

Dr. B: Some schools and organizations offer support groups for siblings of children on the spectrum. To be a sibling of an ASD child certainly carries its own trials. The time involved in meeting the needs of a child with autism may leave exhausted parents with little time for their other children. The siblings may feel the stress of frustration over the enormous time that parents must direct toward the child on the spectrum. They have likely felt some level of embarrassment over the actions of the ASD child in public. The siblings may not feel free to invite friends to the home for fear of the behavior of the child with autism. They often have been the target of aggression by the ASD child having a meltdown. Some tell of being overachievers due to a need to try to make up for the status of the other child. Typical children are sensitive to the stresses their parents are feeling and take on some of that stress. Like their parents, they may have concerns about the future for the sibling. They may worry about their role as a future caregiver. Every child needs the opportunity to feel special to his parents and to know his parents make every effort for equity between the siblings.

Getting children to help with chores around the house may be difficult in even the most compliant children. For children who are not motivated by social approval or praise, it can be more difficult. The expectation becomes more complicated by difficulty following directions, poor sensory processing, and problems sequencing. You may find more success when you break any task into its smallest units and teach the steps. Use the information you have gathered about how your child learns best and what specific sensory issues may interfere with his success.

Elizabeth: At first, your child may not respond, but he will learn. Remember, your child understands much more than he can communicate. Keep it simple if he is not responding to you. Take your child by the hand and help him comply if he will not do it unaided. Transitioning to a new task can be a highly emotional time. Try not to take it personally. Use the hand over hand method to sign (and say) *finished* or *stop* to signal the completion of the task.

Mrs. Nic: Jackie tells me that her son, John, has a fear of germs. He will, however, take out the trash and feed the dog if he is given rubber gloves to wear. I work with another family who feels like new chores are resisted so strongly because as each one is introduced, it is a change to the child's routine. If his routine for years is to get up and leave the table after dinner, then he is suddenly asked to help clear the table, this would be a difficult change for him. If his mom put his freshly washed clothes into his drawers for as long as he can remember, it throws his world into a tailspin if he is now expected to take his folded clothes to the drawers himself.

Mrs. Luck: Remember to use what you know about your child's learning style. Most ASD children learn better visually than through hearing. Visual schedules and visual charts depicting the steps of the task usually help. Show him what you want him to do rather than telling him. Then follow up with visual charts.

Many children on the spectrum will actually keep their own rooms clean without prompting because they have a tendency to prefer an organized, clean environment. He relies on his environment being predictable, consistent, and orderly.

Dr. B: Think of all the time you spend teaching your child and doing his therapies. If you can come up with ways to combine the household tasks with concepts you are teaching, you will be making the most of your time. Your child gets a double benefit. If he helps sort laundry, he is learning colors and vocabulary. A mom I know named Temple tells me that when Tony puts the silverware away, he is working on his matching skills. What a great way to make learning meaningful.

Elizabeth: Social referencing is when a child looks or refers to others to have his accomplishments acknowledged. A child with autism displays little of this behavior. He will accomplish tasks as a means to an end. A child with autism will not usually do an activity to please another person. The child may do it because he is interested, desires the end reward, wishes to avoid consequences, or because he knows it will help end the session if he complies. Social referencing should come as your child progresses, so always encourage it by offering praise and acknowledgement.

Dr. B: The most important thing caregivers do for children is to keep them safe. We make every effort to create a safe environment and to teach our children rules and routines that promote our goal. Parents and teachers must be constantly vigilant in every situation to assure the necessary precautions. The home environment, the school, and the community all hold threats that must be anticipated.

Parents typically baby-proof their homes with baby gates and plastic guards over the electrical outlets. They remove small non-edible objects from a child's view. As the typical child moves through the preschool years, many of the early precautions can be eliminated. Parents of children on the spectrum need to remain highly vigilant for years. The parents may use increased locks for security or limit the access that the child has to certain areas where he may get hurt. Wandering off is one problem behavior, but other children are runners. Many parents use door alarms along with childproof locks if their child tends to be a wanderer or a runner. Since sleep is an issue for many ASD children (and their parents), some families find it necessary to alarm the bedroom doors, so they are alerted if the child leaves his bedroom at night. Some families purchase personal tracking devices using GPS technology that can help to locate their child if he wanders or runs away. If your child is a runner, you will think in terms of safety layers. At home, your interior rooms may have alarms and locks, and so will the exterior doors. If your yard is gated, you will alarm and lock those barriers also. These children become escape artists. They figure out codes and how to unlock locks. If you use locks high on the door above their reach, expect that they will grab a tool to extend their reach and pop the lock. If you use small alarms that attach to the body and are activated as they cross the threshold of a door, they learn to remove those devices. I have seen young children climb over a six-foot-high wooden privacy fence in a split second as the caretaker chases behind. These kids are smart, and they are fast.

Children with more severe autism tend to *elope*, as it is called, more often than those with a less severe diagnosis. Some kids enjoy the chase. They think it is fun to bolt. As they start to run, you will see them look back and smile as the chase begins. Others have a different goal; they are actually trying to get someplace. They have a certain destination in mind.

Mike and Cathy have a nonverbal eight-year-old named Leslie. Les tries to escape from the house at all times of the day or night because he wants to go to the grocery store for candy.

Keeping runners safely contained is an issue at school as well. If your child tends to either wander or run, make sure the school is informed and has precautions in place.

On my first official day as director at the autism center (working for a company that had just purchased the school), I was attending a meeting at the state capital, two hours away. I received a call telling me that eight-year-old Jonas eloped unnoticed. He was picked up running naked a couple of blocks away by a meals-on-wheels lady delivering lunch to local senior citizens. The kind lady gathered him up and called the police. The policeman figured that he had come from our school and brought him back.

I left the meeting I was attending and quickly returned to the school to meet with the policeman and representatives from the child protective services agency. When the officials left, I met with the teachers at the center. They showed me how the child escaped through the front door by quickly pressing buttons to deactivate the door alarm. I immediately called the alarm company and had the system in the building expanded and updated. The cost was minimal for the peace of mind that we were doing all we could to protect the children.

As you look for safety hazards around your home, try to think like your child does. Is he a child who may pick up objects and throw them across the room? Is he a curious little scientist who wants to see what happens when he flushes objects down the toilet or obsessively sticks things into sockets? Consider every safety issue through your own child's eyes. Modify the environment and teach safety through rules and by modeling.

Shelli: It is more difficult to modify the environment outside your home. I had mixed feelings when I first saw websites that sell bright yellow triangular traffic signs cautioning "Autistic Child in Neighborhood" similar to those warning drivers of blind or deaf children in the area. The more I thought about it, the less offended I felt. Safety of the child is the most important factor, and let's face it. We need all the help we can get.

Elizabeth: One positive aspect to home life is the addition of pets. Pets take our time and sometimes our patience. However, let me tell you pets can be so worth every minute you invest in them. I had the glorious idea that I would get a dog and train it to be a therapy dog. Well, our family ended up rescuing two puppies. One of them seemed like she needed therapy herself. Seven years later, they became the perfect therapy dogs. Who was I kidding? I didn't have time to train a dog, let alone two puppies. With that said, there was something I can't deny. From the start, they knew their role in our family. They relentlessly jumped and licked everyone except Nathan. If he approached them they froze, allowing him to pet them. They knew. They knew they had to be still for him. Even as very young puppies, they would not jump on him. The dogs would watch him, waiting until he was finished. They would look at me for confirmation. I would say, "Okay, he is done. Go play." Then they would scamper off.

Today, the dogs offer Nathan so much comfort. They let him sit them up in a human position next to him and watch movies. When I walk in, they look at me with that I-know-you-aren't-going-to-make-me-get-off-the-couch-because-I-am-with-Nathan look. It is a very symbiotic relationship. Yes, it is worth it.

I do caution that the relationship often doesn't look like it does in the movies. See it for what it is for your child. Don't try to fit the mold of the loyal therapy dog. Let the relationship develop. I wanted a dog that would allow the identifying therapy jacket and assist me. Instead, I got a good-old-boy-and-his-dogs relationship, and it couldn't be better.

Mrs. Luck: Kyle is a high school boy who tells me about his pets. His dad wants him to brush the dog, which he will do if he has gloves to wear. He wears the gloves when he walks the dog, in case the need should arise to touch the dog for any reason. His family also has a cat. Kyle's mom says during meals, Kyle gets extremely upset because he thinks the cat stares at him, plotting to steal his food.

Dr. B: Making it through the challenges of day-to-day family life gets even more complicated when a holiday rolls around. Extra responsibilities are felt by the parent. Holiday preparations and celebrations require time and disrupt the routines you have worked so hard to establish.

Shelli: Holidays are characterized by a lot of hustle and bustle, which I have never been a fan of. To me, chaos can steal the joy from the holidays. Crowds, thousands of lights, Christmas trees, family gatherings, all become overwhelming. My husband and I have done our best over the last couple of years to create happy memories for our kids during the holidays.

My advice for Christmas shopping is to try to pick one day to do all the shopping. Find a sitter and leave the kids out of the crazy shopping experiences at all cost. Lines are usually longer during the holidays. This waiting is too much for a lot of kids on the spectrum. Keep it calm. Keep it happy.

When our children were small, we would make an effort to please everyone in the extended family. We would go to Thanksgiving dinners and Christmas celebrations with every branch of our relatives. We would visit his grandparents, my grandparents (both sides), his mom and dad, my mom and dad, and then celebrate at our own house. This would mean that on holidays, we were on the go all day or weekend long. Each place would have different expectations for the kids. This was not fun for the kids or for us as parents. Now on Thanksgiving, if the family dinner is not being hosted at our house, then we only go to one place. We stay as long as the kids can handle it, and then we leave. We don't try to push the kids.

During the Christmas holidays, car rides have been our favorite tradition with the kids. We drive around to various neighborhoods and look at the Christmas lights. Our kids love it. We pack peppermint sticks and drinks in the car. Since the whole activity takes place in the car, there is no chance of a child running off or getting into something that they should not. I can relax in that knowledge. It is fun for all of us. They are buckled in and restrained, yet there is enough stimulation to keep them satisfied. I think it makes them happy that it is just our family, and there are no strangers to approach them. It is the perfect activity for children like mine.

Opening gifts is so much fun. It can get crazy with paper everywhere, family laughing, and crowded spaces. Keep in mind that it can all get overwhelming for someone on the spectrum. My advice is to take it slowly. If you are away from home, ask the host if there is a room you can retreat to if a break is needed. Bring a book or some paper and crayons that your kids can take with them to the quiet area. If they need to work out their jitters ask about a trampoline or a swing set. Bundle up and go outside for a moment. Let your kids be themselves. Think ahead. Control the environment as much as you can. If you and your children become stressed, say your good-byes. You can always open gifts later. You could take pictures or video the children opening the gifts and send it to the giver along with a thank-you note. This is better than everyone being stressed. If your host is not flexible with you or not willing to accommodate your child's needs, just mark them off the list of places to visit on the holidays for now. I know that we all worry about hurting people's feelings, especially during the holidays, but we have to look at what is best for our family. If they want you to be a part of the celebration, they will make adjustments.

Christmas is a big deal to me, and I really like to make it wonderful for our children. We stay at home for Christmas Day. We wear our PJs, and we eat breakfast when the kids are ready. We open gifts when the kids are ready. We don't open them all at once. If my kids want to just play with the boxes instead of the toys, that is okay. If my house gets trashed it's okay too. We have pillow fights and read books and laugh together. My family can come to us if they want, but I'm in charge at my house, so I have more control. This seems to work for us. You will know what will work for you. Plan ahead. Prepare.

Through the holidays, make picture schedules to help your kids know what is next. My kids like predictability, and I can control that more when we are in our own home. When we go to places where people don't have kids like ours, they don't grasp the extreme importance of knowing what comes next. Staying home takes a lot of the stress out of the holidays.

Birthdays are fun. They are all about the birthday boy or girl. I don't like to tell friends we are having a birthday party because they tend to expect the traditional birthday routines—sit down for cake and ice cream, and open gifts with everyone looking at you. No, no! My kids hate this activity. I like to just invite friends to get together, and we just relax and let the kids play. My family will ask for suggestions on what to get the children for their birthdays. They frown if I tell them things like lotion, shaving cream (for sensory activities), finger paints, and bubbles. These things will make my kids happy. We go through a lot of shampoo, shaving cream, and lotion in our home. My kids love rubbing their hands through those products. When I pull these items out, I know I can get the dishes done without interruption or get the laundry folded without it being unfolded before I can get it put away. Toys don't pull rank in my home. A new doll or some other toy quickly loses the popularity contest. This is just the way it is.

Holiday decorations can be a challenge. First of all, our kids don't like change, so they don't really want the decorations put up at all. Christmas season smells different, looks different, and sounds different than the rest of the year. It even tastes different, with Christmas foods appearing on the table. And the music, no thanks. So we either start really early in the season, get sneaky, and put up a tiny bit at a time, hoping they don't notice, or we do it all very quickly right at the last minute, like ripping off a Band-Aid.

Mrs. Luck: As soon as the tree goes up, a lot of my children think they should get to open presents that very minute. A calendar where you can mark off the days until December 25 will be helpful. They do not understand the wait. Keep reminding yourself that our children perceive auditory and visual stimuli differently than other people do. I knew a little boy whose favorite activity during the holidays was to lie *under* the Christmas tree and look up through it. He had his own unique way of enjoying the tree.

Relationships

Dr. B: The task of raising a family brings both joys and challenges. When one or more members of the family have special needs, the challenges are multiplied. When the family member has autism, tensions can be magnified. The more severe the level of autism, the more attention the child will require, and the more the entire family life revolves around that child. Medical and educational costs are astronomical, adding to the family stress. Lack of sleep makes coping more difficult.

Following normal marital advice seems to be easier said than done for families with children on the spectrum. You frequently hear that having a regular "date night" is healthy for a marriage, and parents should take time to be alone as a couple. Making those arrangements may be next to impossible in many situations. Family dynamics are difficult and maintaining healthy relationships demands time and energy. Parents of special needs children have a higher than average divorce rate. Studies show that most divorced couples who have an offspring on the spectrum do not blame the autism itself for the breakup. However, all the related baggage the diagnosis carries certainly changes parental relationships.

Although people on the spectrum often have trouble developing and maintaining relationships, friendships are an important part of a healthy adult life. It can take a great deal of time and guidance for people with autism to form relationships with family members and friends. It will not come naturally. It must be encouraged and taught.

Mrs. Luck: A student walked into my room two years ago and announced, "I hate speech and I hate you." On the last day of school this year, she stopped by to see me, we talked awhile, and then she asked if she could give me a hug. It was a very sweet moment. It had taken a long time and a lot of work, but it was certainly worth it.

Dr. B: Parents of children on the spectrum generally feel judged by others. Most likely, people are indeed judgmental until they are informed and educated about autism and Asperger's syndrome. An uninformed observer watching behavior that is outside his level of acceptance may just think this is a misbehaving child. Behaviors associated with autism can be easily misjudged as bad parenting. When they see a child screaming in the local convenience store, they think he should be spanked. If they see a youngster banging his head in the grocery store, they may think he is throwing a temper tantrum and simply should be punished.

Too many people do not understand the first thing about autism. Those people may even make rude or insensitive comments about the behaviors they see. People may stare. Have a plan when you go out in public. Understand the types of situations that can upset your child and do your best to avoid these circumstances whenever possible.

It would be a monumental task to inform people about autism one by one. But we chip away at the public ignorance on the topic. Get involved with larger groups of people who are raising awareness of autism. Work with organizations who promote education about ASD. We have to make information available to people if we expect them to understand. The future of our society depends on it.

Final Thoughts

Elizabeth: As I write my final thoughts for this project, I pause to sing to a child who requested a lullaby. My mind is distracted as I think of my father's bypass surgery in the morning. I remember that above all I am a mother, a wife, a daughter, a sister, and a friend. Autism is a part of my life. Just like these relationships, I have a relationship with autism. It is an intimate relationship that I am bound to through love. While autism does not define my children, it is a part of them. I love them, not despite their autism but including their autism.

If you ask me to look at the bright side of autism I can. There are some perks to this diagnosis. Year after year, hearing each muted "I love you" is like hearing it for the first time. Grand accomplishments come in small steps. Make-believe never ends. Trying to capture leprechauns is a yearly event. Simple is preferred. Organization is vital. Bravery is common. And love is unbiased.

My hope is that as families journey with autism they always see their child first. That they help them pursue their talents, capture their gifts, and develop their character. Whether it be voice acting, teaching, or putting together puzzles, help your children find joy in what they do and rejoice in their achievements. It is an amazing journey. Don't miss it because you forgot to enjoy the ride.

Shelli: I hope you enjoyed reading this book as much as we enjoyed writing it. My final advice to you is to look every day for those things that your kids are good at. Focus on what they do well. Be excited about their victories. No matter how small the accomplishment is, it matters. Celebrating each achievement will be good medicine for you, and it will be the driving force that will pave the path of success for your *totally amazing kid*. You hold the key to your child's success. I wish you and your family the very best of luck.

Mrs. Nic: As a classroom teacher, it is very difficult to anticipate the needs of each child entering your classroom. We can, however, look at statistics and know that the odds are great that we will at some time have a child on the autism spectrum. In early education, it is our duty to be as knowledgeable as possible about autism, both to use best practices when teaching this child, and also to be open to the possibility that we may have a child not yet diagnosed. Many of the ideas proposed in this book can also be adapted to students not on the autism spectrum, but having other needs. Knowledge is power, and we need all the power we can get to help our students achieve their maximum potential.

My final thoughts to you are about *fear*. To the parents: I urge you not to fear the diagnosis. To have a confirmed diagnosis is your path to early intervention and your source for some funding. I urge you not to be afraid to have expectations of your children. I ask you not to resist working with your child due to fear of the meltdown.

To the teachers: I urge you not to fear working with children on the spectrum. These children are simply *that*: children. They are little human beings fighting to make their way in a world that is topsy-turvy to them. Don't be afraid to get to know this person as an individual, not just as a special needs label. Don't be afraid to have this student in your class. Don't be afraid of the meltdowns. They will happen. You will deal with it and move forward. Don't be afraid to step out of your comfort zone and teach this child in a completely different way than you have taught before. He can make you cry, but at other times, he can really make you laugh. And finally, don't be afraid to just really let yourself enjoy each child.

Mrs. Luck: My final advice is for everyone who deals in any capacity with a child on the spectrum. Love them for what they are, forgive them for what they are not, and teach them all you can. Look beyond the label. The diagnosis does not define the child; it is just one aspect of him. Acceptance is a process. Through acceptance we can best help each one meet the goal of being a happy, productive person. We want to help develop the child's maximum potential of contributing to society and being self-sufficient financially and socially.

Be dedicated to stretching each child's social skills. Gently bring him to the edge of his comfort zone, go a tiny bit further, and then ease back. Do this on a consistent basis, and he will slowly gain the skills necessary to lead a better more fulfilled life. If you do not stretch his skills, the student will retreat into a smaller tighter circle of behaviors that will not benefit him or your family. My final words to you are: *love*, *forgive*, and *teach*. But that's no different than our advice concerning *all* children, is it?

Dr. B: Years ago, when autism was rarely heard of, it didn't really matter whether the general public understood the challenges and characteristics. Just a few decades ago, most people would go through life, never knowing a person on the spectrum. Times have changed. Now as a society, we must understand autism and together support the social, educational, and medical needs of this population. Even though *autism* is now a household word, many people do not understand the first thing about it.

We hope that our words provide insight and understanding. There are topics in this book that all the authors agree upon, such as the importance of early intervention. There are other subjects where you read our differences of opinion. But at the root of everything each of us wrote is a profound respect for the parents and teachers who are faced with enormous challenges.

For the larger community, education is the only avenue to autism awareness. Understanding does not come quickly, as it is a complex disorder. It falls to those of us who live in a world touched by autism to enlighten those on the outside peeking in. Whether you are a parent, teacher, student or friend, you can spread the information that will educate the world about autism.

I mentioned in the Introduction that Muse Watson inspired us to write this book. He encouraged each parent and teacher to reach out to others and share our stories. He reminded us that unmet goals do not mean we have failed; they just mean that we have not yet succeeded.

Rabbi Harold Kushner said, "The purpose of life is to grow and share."[22] We hope that the words we have shared with you will give you a smile, some new ideas, and comfort in the knowledge that you are not on this journey alone.

Suggested Readings

D r. B: If you are inspired to read more on the topic of autism, these are some of the books that we particularly like. The gold standard textbook is *Autism Spectrum Disorders: Issues in Assessment and Intervention* by Patricia Prelock.[23] If you want to invest in a resource for the academic reader, this comprehensive book includes detailed studies and is a great reference tool.

Each of the authors of *Stars in Her Eyes* has chosen a book that she would like to recommend to you. For a reader friendly book, I think you would like *A Regular Guy Growing Up With Autism: A Family's Story of Love and Acceptance,* by Laura Shumaker.[24] This book is my pick for you. It follows one family's journey through life with an autistic son. This is a heart-warming short easy read chronicling milestones in the life of one boy.

Mrs. Nic: *Understanding Autism for Dummies*[25] is a general reference book written by Stephen Shore, who is an adult with autism. Shore offers bullet point personal perspectives on autism, as well as including stories by others who also offer personal experiences. He gives brief, quick explanations of autism from his personal point of view. It is a very basic book, but does include a great amount of information about controversial treatments such as biomedical treatments and nutrition therapy. Much of the book focuses on adults with autism. I suggest this book for you.

Mrs. Luck: *Thinking in Pictures; My Life with Autism,* by Temple Grandin, PhD[26] is a powerful description of the life of an absolutely brilliant woman who has autism, yet becomes an accomplished author, lecturer and animal scientist. This book is my pick for you. The movies chronicling the life of Temple Grandin are also inspiring.

Shelli: *The Out-of-Synch Child,* by Carol Stock Kranowitz[27], which is a popular book in the autism community is my pick for you. This book focuses on sensory processing difficulties and the remediation of that disorder to help children on the autism spectrum. It includes adaptable fun activities to increase sensory processing skills. Written in easy to understand terms, it is applicable to the younger, lower functioning child.

Elizabeth: My pick for you is *Now I See the Moon,* by Elaine Hall.[28] As parents we have little time for free reading. That is why I thoroughly enjoy Elaine's book. It is informative and inspiring, yet it reads like a novel. When I read it I feel like I am doing something for myself. I crawl in bed and look forward to my chapter that night.

Dr. B: If you prefer short fast reading material, look for blogs and facebook pages. I personally follow about a dozen autism or therapy pages every day. My favorite is the facebook page *You Know You Have a Child with Autism When...* It is a light hearted, uplifting page where families share positive messages and note their children's successes. There are other facebook pages where people go to vent, and that idea serves a need and has its place.

Elizabeth and Shelli both write their own blogs which I invite you to share. Elizabeth's blog, *TheBailiwickProject. blogspot.com,* allows you to glimpse her amazing life. Shelli's blog page titled *ThatAutismMom.com* is lovingly dedicated to helping others who struggle with the daily trials and treats of living with children with autism.

Elizabeth: I am suggesting four more blogs you may enjoy. I read each of these regularly.

www.idoinautismland.blogspot.com. This blog gives us great insight into the world of autism by one who lives it. Unable to communicate verbally, Ido has no loss of words as he teaches us what autism really means to him.

www.lovethatmax.com. This blog is the portal to special needs blogging. The author engages the community to share their experiences and thoughts.

www.autism-light.blogspot.com. A father of a young boy with autism brings us a blog packed with information and sources. It might just become your "go to" blog.

www.autism-blog.com. Autism Blogger is an entire online support group, but also allows for spreading the word about supports and connects you to others bloggers.

Dr. B: Many local or state communities have their own communication tools. In our area, we enjoy Dayna Busch-Ault's monthly Missouri Autism Report, a magazine which is now available on line as well as in print form.

Finding good resources that you personally relate to is like a treasure hunt. Through your readings you will not only gain knowledge, but you will also begin to feel the arms of others wrapping around you in support.

Bibliography

1. "Data and Statistics." www.cdc.gov/ncbddd/autism/data.

2. "Early Intervention." www.autism-society.org/living-with-autism.

3. "Data and Statistics." www.cdc.gov/ncvddd/autism/data.

4. "Autism Study in South Korea Finds Higher Rate." *Huffington Post*, 2011. www.HuffingtonPost.com/2011/autism-study-South-Korea.

5. Leo Kanner. "Autistic Disturbances of Affective Contact," *Nervous Child*, 2 (1943): 217-250,

6. Jenny McCarthy. "The Doctors TV." www.thedoctorstv.com/main/content/Jenny_Mccarthy_Autism.

7. S. Santangelo, and S. Folstein. *The Genetics of Autism in: Neurodevelopmental Disorders*, (MA: MIT Press, 1999), 431-447.

8. Autism Society, "Early Intervention." www.autism-society.org/living-with-autism.

9. "Stephen Shore." http://www.myinfinitec.org/resources/autism.

10. "The Picture Exchange Communication System." http:www.autism-society.org/living-with-autism/treatment-options/pecs.

11. J. Piaget. *Play, Dreams, and Imitation in Childhood.* Trans. C. Gattegno and Hodgson, F. M. (New York: W.W. Norton & Company, 1962).

12. "Dragons Kicker with Autism Redefines Special Needs." http:www.Brick.patch.com.

13. Stephanie Wilkerson. "Assessing Teacher Attitude Toward the Inclusion of Students with Autism," *PhD Diss., University of Louisville.*

14. Golnik, A, M. Ireland, and I. Borowsky. "Medical Homes for Children with Autism: A Physician Survey." *Official Journal of the American Academy of Pediatrics.* (2013).

15. Autism Speaks, "Tool Kits- Dentist Guide." http:www.AutismSpeaks.org/familyservices/tool-kits.

16. Autism Speaks, "Tool Kits- Emergency Information Packet." http:www.AutismSpeaks.org/familyservices/tool-kits.

17. Interactive Autism Network, www.iancommunity.org/cs/glossary_term?glossary.id=271.

18. MacDonald, M. "Autistic Children with Better Motor Skills More Adept at Socializing." *Science Daily*, 2013.

19. The Gray Center, "Social Stories." http:www.Thegray center.org/socialstories.

20. "Declaration of Presence of FD&C YellowNo.5." www.law.cornell.edu/cfr/text/21/201.20.

21. J. Humphreys, P. Gringas, P. Blair, N. Scott, J. Henderson, P. Fleming, and A. Edmond. "Sleep Patterns in Children with Autistic Spectrum Disorders: a prospective cohort study." *Archives of Disease in Childhood* (2013).

22. "Harold S. Kushner." http:www.goodreads.com/ quote.

23. Patricia Prelock. *Autism Spectrum Disorders: Issues in Assessment and Intervention*, (Austin, Texas: Pro Ed, 2006).

24. Laura Shumaker. *A Regular Guy Growing Up with Autism*, (Sherwood, OR: Landscape Press, 2008).

25. Stephen Shore, and L. Rastelli. *Understanding Autism for Dummies*, (New York: Wiley, John and Sons, Inc, 2011).

26. Temple Grandin. *Thinking in Pictures; My Life with Autism*, (New York: Knopf Doubleday Publishing, 2010).

27. Carol Kranowitz. *The Out of Synch Child*, (USA: Penguin Press, 2006).

28. Elaine Hall. *Now I See the Moon*, (New York: Harper Collins, 2010).